NO AR

S0-AEE-017

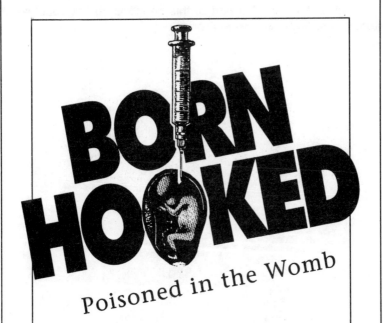

Poisoned in the Womb

New Revised
Second Edition

IDEAS in CONFLICT

Gary E. McCuen

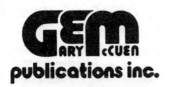

publications inc.

411 Mallalieu Drive
Hudson, Wisconsin 54016
Phone (715) 386-7113

Illustrations and Photo Credits

Engage/Social Action 53, 62, 67, 93, General Accounting Office 21, 29, 100, David Horsey 105, Dick Locher 139, Craig MacIntosh 81, *St. Paul Pioneer Press* 42, 47, David Seavey 128, 133, U.S. Department of Health and Human Services 11, *Wisconsin State Journal* 16, Richard Wright 87

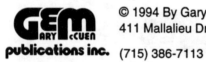

© 1994 By Gary E. McCuen Publications, Inc.
411 Mallalieu Drive, Hudson, Wisconsin 54016

(715) 386-7113

International Standard Book Number
0-86596-091-7
Printed in the United States of America

CONTENTS

Chapter 3 **FETAL NEGLECT AND SOCIAL RESPONSE**

Chapter 4 CRIME, PREGNANCY AND DRUGS

REASONING SKILL DEVELOPMENT

These activities may be used as individualized study guides for students in libraries and resource centers or as discussion catalysts in small group and classroom discussions.

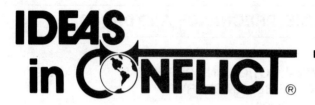

IDEAS in CONFLICT ®

This series features ideas in conflict on political, social, and moral issues. It presents counterpoints, debates, opinions, commentary, and analysis for use in libraries and classrooms. Each title in the series uses one or more of the following basic elements:

Introductions that present an issue overview giving historic background and/or a description of the controversy.

Counterpoints and debates carefully chosen from publications, books, and position papers on the political right and left to help librarians and teachers respond to requests that treatment of public issues be fair and balanced.

Symposiums and forums that go beyond debates that can polarize and oversimplify. These present commentary from across the political spectrum that reflect how complex issues attract many shades of opinion.

A *global* emphasis with foreign perspectives and surveys on various moral questions and political issues that will help readers to place subject matter in a less culture-bound and ethnocentric frame of reference. In an ever-shrinking and interdependent world, understanding and cooperation are essential. Many issues are global in nature and can be effectively dealt with only by common efforts and international understanding.

Reasoning skill study guides and discussion activities provide ready-made tools for helping with critical reading and evaluation of content. The guides and activities deal with one or more of the following:

RECOGNIZING AUTHOR'S POINT OF VIEW

INTERPRETING EDITORIAL CARTOONS

VALUES IN CONFLICT

WHAT IS EDITORIAL BIAS?

WHAT IS SEX BIAS?

WHAT IS POLITICAL BIAS?

WHAT IS ETHNOCENTRIC BIAS?

WHAT IS RACE BIAS?

WHAT IS RELIGIOUS BIAS?

*From across **the political spectrum** varied sources are presented for research projects and classroom discussions. Diverse opinions in the series come from magazines, newspapers, syndicated columnists, books, political speeches, foreign nations, and position papers by corporations and nonprofit institutions.*

About the Editor

Gary E. McCuen is an editor and publisher of anthologies for public libraries and curriculum materials for schools. Over the past years his publications have specialized in social, moral and political conflict. They include books, pamphlets, cassettes, tabloids, filmstrips and simulation games, many of them designed from his curriculums during 11 years of teaching junior and senior high school social studies. At present he is the editor and publisher of the *Ideas in Conflict* series and the *Editorial Forum* series.

CHAPTER 1

POISONED IN THE WOMB: AN OVERVIEW

1

POISONED IN THE WOMB:
AN OVERVIEW

BOARDER BABIES AND
ABANDONED INFANTS

U.S. Dept. of Health and Human Services

The following article is excerpted from the report entitled, "National Estimates on the Number of Boarder Babies, the Cost of Their Care, and the Number of Abandoned Infants". It is based on data gathered and analyzed under a study which provided the Department of Health and Human Services the information necessary to determine the estimated number of boarder babies residing in hospitals nationwide. The study further examined the number and characteristics of infants who were not yet medically ready for discharge from the hospital, but who would most likely be placed by a child welfare agency in the custody of someone other than their biological parent(s).

Points to Consider:

1. Define the purpose of the Abandoned Infants Assistance Act.

2. What kind of study does this act require?

3. How are boarder babies distinguished from abandoned infants?

4. Why is drug use related to the health of these babies?

Excerpted from a report to Congress titled "National Estimates on the Number of Boarder Babies and Abandoned Infants" by the U.S. Department of Health and Human Services, August 1993.

*Three-fourths of the boarder babies and two thirds
of the abandoned infants are African American.*

The Abandoned Infants Assistance Act of 1988 (Pub. L. 100-505, as amended) was enacted by Congress to assist States in addressing the problem of an increasing number of infants residing in hospitals whose parents are unable or unwilling to provide care at the time the infants are medically ready to be discharged from the hospital. The law was enacted in response to concerns that infants who were medically ready for discharge were remaining in hospitals for days, and sometimes months, while child welfare agencies endeavored to find alternative placements for these infants or provide the in-home services necessary to permit the infant to remain safely in the care of the biological parent(s).

BOARDER BABIES

These infants, who are frequently referred to as "boarder babies", created new demands on the already scarce resources available to child welfare agencies and hospitals, particularly in poor, urban areas. Many of these infants were reported to be born to mothers who had been using crack/cocaine during their pregnancy, and some were also reported to have tested positive for the human immunodeficiency virus (HIV). In addition, many of these infants were born prematurely, had low birthweights, or had medical problems that required specialized care. Not only are children who remain in the hospital beyond the point of medical need deprived of the opportunity to grow and develop in a nurturing environment, but medically unnecessary hospital care for these children also results in additional costs and a drain on limited medical resources when care in a non-institutional setting would be more appropriate.

In an attempt to remedy this problem, the Abandoned Infants Assistance Act authorized funding for grants to public and non-profit private entities for the purpose of developing, implementing, and operating programs to demonstrate methods of serving abandoned infants and young children, especially those with acquired immune deficiency syndrome (AIDS).

HEALTH AND HUMAN SERVICES STUDY

In addition, the law, as amended, requires that the Secretary of the Department of Health and Human Services conduct a study for the purpose of determining:

10

(A) an estimate of the number of infants and young children abandoned in hospitals in the United States and the number of such infants who are infected with HIV or who have been perinatally exposed to the virus or who have been perinatally exposed to a dangerous drug;

(B) an estimate of the annual costs incurred by the Federal Government and by state and local governments in providing housing and care for such infants and young children. P.L. 100-505, Section 102 (c) (1) and (2).

This study examined the numbers and characteristics of both

"boarder babies" and "abandoned infants". For purposes here, "boarder babies" are defined as infants, under 12 months of age, who remain in the hospital beyond the date of medical discharge. They may eventually be released to the care of their biological parent(s) or placed in an alternative care setting. "Abandoned infants" are defined as infants, under 12 months of age, who are unlikely to leave the hospital in the custody of their biological parent(s) once they are discharged. This includes infants whom the child welfare agency believes cannot safely remain in the care of their biological parent(s) as well as infants whose parent(s) are unwilling or unable to provide care.

Findings from the study included:

Boarder Babies

At one time during calendar year 1991, there were 10,000 boarder babies residing in 573 hospitals throughout 101 counties in the United States. Boarder babies who were in the hospital on the census day had a median length of stay of seven days prior to medical discharge and a median length of stay of five days after medical discharge up until the census day. Sixty-five percent of the boarder babies stayed less than ten days beyond their medical discharge until the census day; while almost one-fourth (24 percent) stayed from 21 to over 100 days beyond medical discharge until the census day.

The average cost of care per boarder baby is estimated to be $2,930 for five days, the median length of stay past medical discharge, and $12,892 for 22 days, the mean length of stay past medical discharge. These estimated costs are based on the inclusive rates provided by hospitals and included the board rate plus ancillary charges (e.g. the use of an apnea monitor or fees for laboratory tests).

The annual minimum cost of the care of boarder babies is estimated to be $22.3 million using the median of five days stay beyond medical discharge and based on actual hospital rates. The maximum estimated annual cost is $125 million using the mean length of stay of 22 days beyond medical discharge and based on costs only from hospitals providing inclusive rates, that is, the board rate plus ancillary charges.

Abandoned Infants

• At some time during calendar year 1991, there were at least

12

12,000 abandoned infants.

- The characteristics of boarder babies and abandoned infants are quite similar.

- Three-fourths of the boarder babies and two-thirds of the abandoned infants are African American.

- Over three-fourths of the boarder babies and abandoned infants who were tested were found to be drug-exposed. Drug exposure could be determined for 74 percent of the boarder babies and 87 percent of the abandoned infants.

- Eight percent of all drug-exposed infants were known to be HIV positive. Sixty-eight percent of all drug-exposed infants were either not tested or had an unknown HIV status.

Placement Arrangements

Slightly over 60 percent of the boarder babies were not expected to leave the hospital with their custodial parent(s). Fifty-five percent of all boarder babies were expected to be placed in family foster homes. Only 2.5 percent were expected to go directly into adoptive home placement.

None of the abandoned infants were expected to leave the hospital in the care of their biological parent(s). Fifty-four percent of the abandoned infants were expected to be placed in foster family care, and six percent were expected to go into adoptive placement.

2

POISONED IN THE WOMB:
AN OVERVIEW

SUBSTANCE ABUSE IN PREGNANCY:
THE ECONOMIC AND SOCIAL COST

Ann Pytkowicz Streissguth, Ph.D.

Ann Pytkowicz Streissguth, Ph.D., is a professor at the Department of Psychiatry and Behavioral Sciences at the University of Washington Medical School. Streissguth specializes in the study of substance abuse during pregnancy.

Points to Consider:

1. Why would it be short-sighted to target prevention programs at only illicit drug use?

2. Why should information dissemination not be limited to only the pregnancy period?

3. Summarize the prognosis of an FAS child.

4. Discuss needed changes in the school to accommodate FAS children.

Excerpted from testimony by Ann Pytkowicz Streissguth before the Senate Committee on Labor and Human Resources, April 11, 1990.

We are facing a national crisis in terms of alcohol and drug abuse during pregnancy.

In understanding the economic and social costs of substance abuse in pregnancy, it is essential that we keep two facts in mind:

1) Illicit drug use among pregnant women is usually accompanied by alcohol use; and

2) Alcohol is a known agent capable of causing life-long disability depending on the pattern and amount consumed.

Therefore, it would be short-sighted to target any intervention/prevention programs at only illicit drug use. When it comes to the fetus, the war on drugs must include both licit and illicit substances of abuse. From the standpoint of adverse effects on the fetus from prenatal exposure, both alcohol and cocaine should be primary targets. However, all substance abuse postnatally can interfere with effective mothering and place the developing child at increased risk of compromised development. Thus both pre- and postnatal substance abuse should be targeted.

PRIMARY PREVENTION

Accelerated programs for primary prevention are urgently needed, not just against illicit drug abuse but against alcohol as well. Larger and more effective bottle labels, warning signs at point of purchase (by drink or by bottle), and restrictive advertising are all urgently needed for alcohol, the drug about which the most is known in terms of long-term damage from prenatal exposure. Of particular importance is dissemination of information about the effects of substance abuse in the period prior to pregnancy recognition. It is often not realized that the baby can be damaged even before the mother realizes she is pregnant. On the other hand, studies also show that stopping alcohol use any time during pregnancy is better for the baby than not stopping at all. Early studies suggest that the same may be true for cocaine abuse as well.

In addition to information dissemination, primary prevention measures should include special drug and alcohol treatment programs for pregnant and postpartum women who are abusing drugs and alcohol, as well as a variety of psychosocial supports to facilitate a healthier lifestyle.

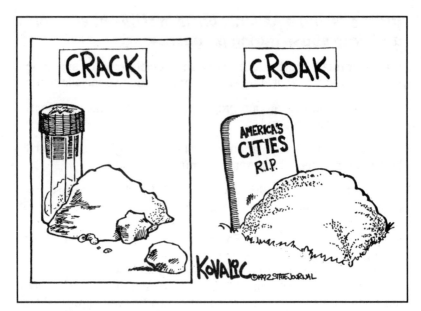

Reprinted by permission of the **Wisconsin State Journal**.

HOW LONG DO THE EFFECTS LAST?

Compared to unexposed children, those who have been drug and cocaine exposed in utero are at a higher risk for developmental deficits during infancy and the earlier preschool years. General developmental milestones as well as emotional and social development appear to be affected. Although long range studies have not yet been carried out, the early signs of disorganized behavior do not bode well for an easy transition into school and the learning and work environment. Funding for long term studies of drug and alcohol exposed children is desperately needed, to understand the nature of the problem and to develop remedial programs.

For alcohol, the consequences of prenatal exposure have been studied across the lifespan in humans and animals. Children diagnosed with Fetal Alcohol Syndrome have a very poor prognosis for independent living even though they may have intellectual development within the normal range. Their prenatal brain damage and the disorganized behavioral patterns associated with it make it increasingly difficult to compete in the workplace, to establish stable and supportive social relationships, and to protect themselves against danger. In our long-term studies, they are disproportionately represented among the homeless, the unwed mothers, and

---

22,000 BABIES ABANDONED

Thousands of babies have been abandoned in their hospital cribs by parents unwilling or unable to take them home, according to a draft report from the Department of Health and Human Services.

They are the tiniest victims of crack cocaine, poverty, homelessness and AIDS, and one of the reasons the number of children in foster care is inching toward 500,000. Researchers counted 22,000 abandoned infants and boarder babies in the nation's hospitals in 1991.

"22,000 Babies Abandoned," **Associated Press,** November 9, 1993

---

the victimized. Despite their dysfunctional lives, over half do not readily qualify for protective environments because their IQ levels are too high. The lack of facilities and appropriate help either in the schools or later for persons disabled by prenatal brain damage from alcohol further compromises their development and decreases their chances for productive living.

The State of Washington estimates 133 persons born per year with the full Fetal Alcohol Syndrome, and at the least two times this number per year with possible Fetal Alcohol Effect. Our recent studies show the latter persons to also suffer from long range disabilities. Figures from State Senator Binkeley in Alaska tags the lifetime cost to the state, of each child born with FAS, at $1.4 million. The costs associated with less definitive risks from prenatal alcohol exposure (hyperactivity, attention deficits, learning disabilities, and associated psychopathologies) are difficult to assess, but they affect educational, social, and medical costs at every level.

SECONDARY PREVENTION: DEVELOPING INTERVENTIONS

While it is clear that the consequences of prenatal alcohol exposure can last a lifetime, we also note that affected adults and adolescents have generally not received appropriate interventions. One of the greatest unmet needs is the development of specialized educational and treatment programs for alcohol and drug

17

exposed offspring of all ages. While preschool programs are easy enough to establish, there is virtually nothing being done at the level of primary or secondary education. Yet in communities where alcohol and drug abuse is high, such children may over-whelm the special education programs. Without recognition and appropriate intervention, such children are at high risk for school drop-out. Due to their increasingly disruptive behavior as they get older, they are also at risk for being expelled from regular pro-grams. Once out of the structured environment, tracking and spe-cial programming become almost impossible. They often end up homeless, estranged from families, living in the shadows of life, trying to work but not being able to, usually not qualified for ser-vices.

We are facing a national crisis in terms of alcohol and drug abuse during pregnancy. While one obvious approach is to focus on primary prevention strategies, we must also begin mobilization of secondary prevention or intervention efforts. Without better remedial interventions than exist now, every child with FAS (and many with FAE) is at serious risk for life-long disabilities. We need immediate funding for research into identification and remediation of affected children. Not every child whose mother takes cocaine or alcohol during pregnancy is affected. Research is desperately needed for identification of those with prenatal brain damage so that research on special programs can be undertaken. Programs for identification and remediation are desperately needed at all developmental stages from infancy to adulthood. Mothers with Fetal Alcohol Syndrome are no better able to protect their children from abuse and victimization than they have been able to protect themselves.

3   POISONED IN THE WOMB: AN OVERVIEW

THE IMPACT OF DRUG ABUSE ON THE WELFARE SYSTEM

Richard L. Jones

Richard L. Jones is the executive director of Boston Children's Services. Jones is the Chair of the Child Welfare League of America, Inc., which is comprised of over 650 public and private child welfare agencies in the United States and Canada. He is also the chair of the National Commission on Chemical Dependency and Child Welfare.

Points to Consider:

1. In which population is drug and alcohol use on the rise?

2. Summarize the effects of alcohol and drug exposure on infants.

3. What is the effect of parental drug involvement on the foster care program?

4. Why are there so few resources available in the child welfare system for prevention and intervention?

Excerpted from testimony by Richard L. Jones before the Human Resources Subcommittee of the Full House Committee on Ways and Means, April 30, 1991.

In one study, 100% of homeless and runaway youth in San Francisco reported polydrug use on a regular basis.

The integrity of family life and the well being of children have been profoundly affected by changes in American society in recent decades. Although some segments of American society have enjoyed an improved standard of living, many other groups have experienced fragmentation of family life, economic instability, poor housing or homelessness, and an inability to access basic health care. The same disparities apply to the use of alcohol and other drugs. Although the general population has moderated its consumption of alcohol and other drugs, surveys reveal that disadvantaged and minority communities are, as a group, engaging in an increased daily and/or chronic use of illicit drugs. Particularly troubling is the significant increase in the number of women of child bearing age who abuse drugs.

As parental alcohol and drug use has continued to rise, there has been an ever-growing increase in the number of infants exposed in utero to various illicit drugs, infants and young children abandoned by their parents, and children who are subjected to abuse or neglect because of parental substance abuse. Infants and children are being referred to the child welfare system in unprecedented numbers. At the same time, there has been a dramatic increase in the number of children entering foster care, many of whom are substantially impaired as a result of parental alcohol and drug use.

The following illustrate the immense problem that parental substance abuse poses:

• Pregnant drug abusers identified today are not typically teens, but instead are in their mid-twenties, and are likely to have one or more children in addition to the identified drug-exposed newborn. Maternal alcohol and other drug use are affecting not only the infants born drug-exposed but siblings who live in family environments in which alcohol and other drugs play a major role.

• As a result of maternal drug use, many infants are born every year exposed to one or more illegal substances. It is widely acknowledged that drug-exposed infants are being undercounted.

• Unprecedented numbers of newborns are at risk of abandonment. Drug-exposed infants and infants who test positive for HIV

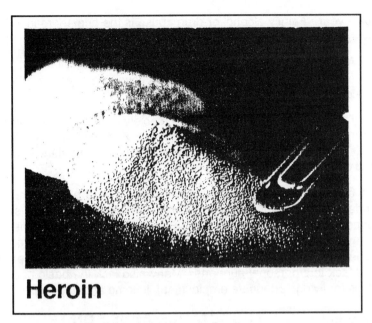

Heroin

Source: General Accounting Office

often remain in the hospital as boarder babies, medically cleared but with no place to go. A Child Welfare League of America one-day survey of five major United States cities discovered that 69% of babies boarding in the surveyed hospitals were born to chemically dependent mothers.

Infants exposed to alcohol and other drugs tend to have complex problems: they are at higher risk of premature birth and low birth weight; are more likely to be affected by Sudden Infant Death Syndrome; tend to display extreme irritability, hypersensitivity to stimulation, excessive crying; have difficulty "bonding" with caregivers; manifest some degree of neurobehavioral deficit; and experience developmental delays. These infants are physically and developmentally fragile.

• Alcohol and drug use may predispose youth to engage in other high risk behaviors, resulting in unintended pregnancies and the spread of sexually transmitted diseases.

• In one study, 100% of homeless and runaway youth in San Francisco reported polydrug use on a regular basis.

• An estimated 1.3 million teens run away or become homeless each year. Family alcohol or drug abuse is the primary reason for over 250,000 of these teens leaving home.

• As many as 40% of the older youth in the child welfare system have had prior juvenile contact, usually involving offenses related to alcohol or drug abuse.

• The costs of substance abuse to society are staggering. It has been estimated that the direct, indirect, and related costs total over $177 billion annually — or about $750 for every man, woman and child in America.

• Chronic use of drugs, especially crack, has been found to undermine an adult's ability to parent. Studies reveal that substance abusing mothers tend to be children of substance abusers themselves, were physically or sexually abused by their parents, suffer from personality disorders of varying degrees of severity, and lack interpersonal supports. Many also lack the basic necessities for living, adequate employment, income and housing.

THE IMPACT OF SUBSTANCE ABUSE ON THE CHILD WELFARE SYSTEM

Given these trends, it is not surprising to find that the child welfare system has been seriously affected by the devastating impact of parental substance abuse on children. The picture is a startling one:

• It is estimated that between 50 and 80 percent of all confirmed child abuse reports and almost three-quarters of child fatalities involve some degree of parental alcohol and/or other drug abuse. Infants and children from chemically involved families are at increased risk of abuse and neglect. Among abused and neglected children, infants are at particularly high risk.

• Alcohol and other drug use have become the predominant characteristic in child protective services caseloads in twenty-two states and the District of Columbia.

• The foster care population, after shrinking in numbers for years, has begun to grow significantly. Drug-exposed infants, toddlers, and preschoolers endangered by parental substance abuse are the fastest growing foster care population.

• The number of very young children in foster care is also growing. Parental drug involvement is believed to be a primary reason

CHILDREN AND WELFARE

The ultimate placement goal for all children in the child welfare system should be a permanent, loving home, either with one's own family or through adoption. Tragically, this is too often not the case today, because the child welfare system is simply overwhelmed.

Shirley E. Marcus, Deputy Director of the Child Welfare League in testimony before the **House Committee on Education**, May 28, 1992

for the foster care placement of these very young children.

• Boarder babies are entering foster care in significant numbers.

• It is estimated that between 30% and 50% of all identified crack-exposed babies enter foster care.

Some experts estimate that up to 80% of drug-exposed infants will be placed in foster care before they reach one year of age. Others suggest that half of the children of addicted women not in treatment programs will enter foster care before they reach a year of age.

OVERWHELMING THE SYSTEM

The escalating number of alcohol and other drug affected children has stressed an overwhelmed child welfare system. Parental substance abuse has made increasing demands on the child welfare system, but at a time when they are most needed, human and fiscal resources within the child welfare system have constricted rather than expanded. The system has been hard pressed to meet its mandate to protect children, preserve families to the maximum extent possible and, when removal is necessary, to reunite children with their families.

The demands on the child welfare system are best appreciated when one considers the system's numerous responsibilities. Child welfare must respond to allegations of abuse or neglect through child protective services; provide crisis services to families at risk of maltreatment or disruption; arrange for out-of-home care when it is in the best interest of the child; provide case management services for children and their families; attempt to reunite children in care with their families; and assure a permanent plan for the child when reunification is not possible. Resources have never been entirely adequate to fully meet these responsibilities but the child welfare system nevertheless managed to hold its own in protecting children and supporting families.

With the dramatic rise in parental substance abuse, however, the system, which was already strained, has reached the breaking point. The unprecedented increase in referrals and the complexity that parental substance abuse introduces into risk assessment and protection of children have placed greater demands on the child welfare system. Child protective service investigations now consume the vast proportion of the human and fiscal resources available to child welfare agencies, and there are few, if any, resources available for prevention, early intervention, and support services, the interventions which vulnerable children and families affected by substance abuse most need to avert a crisis.

WELFARE AGENCIES

Child welfare agencies have encountered numerous obstacles in their efforts to protect children in chemically involved families while simultaneously attempting to assist families in resolving alcohol and drug abuse problems. Many of these obstacles can be characterized as a "lack of": a lack of workers to handle referrals; a lack of training for child welfare professionals regarding substance abuse, addiction, and the impact of substance abuse on parental functioning; a lack of adequate resources to provide the early intervention and support services that alcohol and drug affected families need to ensure the health and well-being of their children; a lack of available, accessible drug treatment, particularly for pregnant and parenting women, the uninsured, and the indigent; a lack of judicial resources that facilitate sound decision-making regarding the needs of children affected by parental substance abuse and the needs of their parents; and a lack of available and appropriate placement options when a child must be removed from parental custody.

As a consequence of these factors, child welfare professionals have experienced frustration and demoralization in their efforts to effectively protect children in chemically dependent families while supporting and enhancing parental functioning. High caseloads have presented a formidable obstacle to early intervention in troubled families. Limited resources have meant that workers are able to address only the most urgent cases and cannot respond to fam-

24

ily problems until they become an emergency. Prevention and early intervention, which clearly offer the greatest probability of success with chemically involved parents, simply cannot be provided because workers must attend to crisis situations in which children are in actual danger or at imminent risk of harm. Moreover, assessment of the risk to the child posed by parental substance abuse has been complicated by inadequate training and supervision and confusing interpretations of what "reasonable efforts" are required to avoid foster care placement of the child.

The child welfare system has been required to assess whether traditional child welfare assessments and interventions are effective with parents who are chemically involved. Workers attempting to provide family focused services are being challenged as never before by parents whose primary or sole interest is obtaining the next supply of drugs. These realities have served to heighten the risk to many vulnerable children, further accentuating the crisis in the child welfare system.

THE INADEQUACY OF DRUG TREATMENT RESOURCES

Further complicating the ability of the child welfare system to respond to the needs of children affected by parental substance abuse and their families is the scarcity of drug treatment resources, particularly for pregnant and parenting women and the uninsured.

The absence of alcohol and drug treatment resources has posed a substantial obstacle to child welfare agencies in their efforts to preserve and strengthen families and to reunite children in out-of-home care with their families. Culturally relevant community-based prevention programs for substance abuse are wholly inadequate. Permanency planning has become difficult, if not impossible, when there are no resources for alcohol and drug treatment which are appropriate for parents who recognize the need for treatment and are motivated to obtain the treatment they need.

4   POISONED IN THE WOMB: AN OVERVIEW

DRUG ADDICTED MOTHERS AND PRENATAL CARE

National Commission to Prevent Infant Mortality

Lawton Chiles, U.S. Senate (Ret.), chaired the National Commission to Prevent Infant Mortality. Chiles is currently serving as Governor of Florida. The following article is an excerpt from the Commission's report.

Points to Consider:

1. Summarize recent statistics on the infant mortality rate in the United States.

2. What are the main risk factors for low birthweight and infant mortality?

3. How would the elimination of maternal smoking affect infant health?

4. What role might family planning have in infant health?

Excerpted from "The National Commission to Prevent Infant Mortality," February, 1990.

Today's topic is one of the most tragic and intractable facets of this nation's drug crisis. Children who were exposed to drugs in the womb face a myriad of challenges; so does the society into which they emerge.

After two decades of steady improvement in infant mortality in the United States, the 1980s came as a shock. Progress in reducing the infant mortality rate stalled, resigning the United States to a rank behind nineteen other developed countries in the rate of infant deaths. The gap between white and black infant death rates widened, leaving black infants more than twice as likely to die in infancy as white infants. Progress in lowering the percentage of infants born with low birthweight stagnated, placing more than one-quarter million infants per year at risk for chronic handicapping conditions. The 1980s also witnessed a growing percentage of women receiving late or no prenatal care, despite the known importance of prenatal care in improving birth outcomes. . .

INFANT DEATHS

The infant mortality rate is an important and sensitive gauge of the health and welfare of a population. Of the 3.8 million infants born in the United States in 1987, nearly 39,000 died before reaching age one, amounting to an infant mortality rate of 10.1 infant deaths per one thousand live births.

At present, the United States ranks a poor twentieth among the developed countries in its infant mortality rate, well behind other nations which, years ago, fared much worse than the United States. Many communities across the country have become infant mortality "disaster areas" — with high rates of infant mortality caused by rampant poverty, unemployment, drug use, and a lack of health care providers.

In order to understand the stalled progress in infant mortality, it is helpful to examine the nature and causes of infant deaths. Infant deaths are usually divided into two categories according to age: neonatal and postneonatal. Neonatal mortality (deaths to infants under 28 days) is generally associated with influences surrounding the pregnancy and birth such as low birthweight, inadequate maternal nutrition, lack of access to prenatal health services, and congenital defects. Postneonatal mortality (deaths to infants between 28 days and one year of age) tends to be associated with the infant's environmental circumstances such as poverty, lack of access to pediatric care, and inadequate food, sanitation, or supervision.

RISK FACTORS

Many of the risk factors for low birthweight and infant mortality have already been identified. Children born to women who are poor, young, minority, under-educated, and those born to women who fail to get early prenatal care or whose pregnancies are unintended are at greatest risk. Increases during the 1980s in "crack" cocaine use, AIDS, syphilis, and births to unmarried mothers further threaten the health of our future generations. Our nation is losing the fight against low birthweight and infant mortality because it has failed to reduce the risks that put the health of mothers and children in jeopardy; in some cases these risks have actually increased.

The problem of crack-addicted pregnant women is recent and escalating. The consequences to the fetus are often serious. Rather than operating as a wall to protect the developing embryo and fetus, the placenta acts more like a sieve, admitting drugs readily from the maternal to the fetal blood stream. Infants born to women who used illegal drugs during pregnancy experience a greater likelihood of prematurity, low birthweight, and congenital defects. They may also suffer from drug withdrawal, and developmental and learning disabilities. Maternal drug use creates an enormous burden for society in its impact on children — yet shockingly few programs exist to treat substance-abusing pregnant women.

Increases in crack use, AIDS, syphilis, and births to unmarried mothers pose immediate threats to infants born in the 1980s, but attention to these problems should not overshadow other well-known behavioral risks which comprise a large portion of preventable infant mortality. Risky behaviors such as smoking and alcohol abuse during pregnancy are strongly associated with poor birth outcomes.

Teen pregnancy is another risk factor which continues to pose a serious threat to the approximately 470,000 babies born to teen mothers each year. Infants born to teen mothers are two to three times more likely to be born with low birthweight. However, the higher rates of infant death and disability are not a foregone conclusion. Teens who receive good prenatal care do not have high-

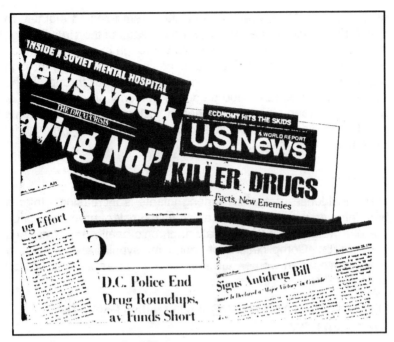

Source: General Accounting Office

er rates of low birthweight or infant mortality. . .

ILLEGAL DRUG USE

Illegal drug use during pregnancy is associated with poor pregnancy outcomes and infant health and development problems. Cocaine use during pregnancy increases the rate of spontaneous abortion, placental abruption, low birthweight, neurobehavioral problems, Sudden Infant Death Syndrome (SIDS), and genitourinary tract malformations.

The incidence of drug abuse during pregnancy among middle- and upper-income women is widely underestimated. A 1989 study found no significant difference between the rate of drug use among women receiving care at public clinics and those visiting private physicians. It also revealed that white women were slightly more likely to abuse drugs during pregnancy than black women.

AIDS

Experts estimate that 30 to 40 percent of the babies born to HIV-infected mothers will go on to develop the disease. Evidence suggests that the AIDS virus is transmitted from infected mothers to their infants while in the uterus by the passage of the virus through the placenta, during labor and delivery through exposure to infected maternal blood and/or vaginal secretions, and, rarely, through breast feeding. The remainder of infections occur through blood transfusions or use of blood products. Minority children, many of whom face urban poverty, poor health, lack of access to adequate health care, and educational disadvantages, comprise the majority of pediatric AIDS cases.

SYPHILIS

The incidence of syphilis among infants is increasing. Infants born infected with syphilis are at increased risk of premature birth, low birthweight, mental retardation, chronic health problems, and early death. Complications of congenital syphilis are completely preventable when women are appropriately screened and treated during pregnancy.

UNMARRIED MOTHERS AND UNINTENDED PREGNANCY

Unmarried mothers are more than three times as likely as married mothers to receive inadequate prenatal care. Infants who are unplanned or unwanted have a greater risk of low birthweight. If all pregnancies were planned, the rate of low birthweight could be reduced by 5 percent among white infants, 16 percent among black infants, and 1 percent overall.

Infant mortality could be reduced an estimated 10 percent if all women not desiring pregnancy used contraception. Family planning is a key program in the effort to reduce infant mortality, prevent teen pregnancy, and halt the spread of AIDS.

SMOKING

Maternal smoking increases the risk of low birthweight births. If maternal smoking were eliminated, we could expect a 25 percent reduction in low birthweight births and a 10 percent reduction in infant mortality. Passive smoking affects infant health. There is a two-fold increase in the incidence of respiratory disease among infants of mothers who smoke, an increase in related hospitalizations, and an increase in Sudden Infant Death Syndrome.

Smoking cessation programs targeted to expectant mothers can significantly increase the birthweight of the baby. These programs achieve 12 to 16 percent higher quit rates than if pregnant women attempt to quit on their own. The Centers for Disease Control estimate that each $1 spent on smoking cessation programs for pregnant women could save $5 on the cost of hospital care for low birthweight infants.

ALCOHOL

Maternal drinking, especially heavy drinking, is associated with miscarriage, mental retardation of the child, low birthweight, and a cluster of congenital defects including nervous system dysfunction called Fetal Alcohol Syndrome (FAS). There is no established safe level of alcohol consumption during pregnancy.

The incidence of Fetal Alcohol Syndrome is estimated at 1 to 3 per 1,000 live births. Among some Native American groups the rate is as high as 10 per 1,000. However, for every child born with FAS, ten times more suffer from alcohol-related problems. Effects can be seen in as many as two-thirds of infants born to women who drink heavily.

Alcohol abuse is a major preventable cause of low birthweight among infants, and the primary preventable cause of mental retardation.

TEEN PREGNANCY

The higher than average infant mortality rate for teens is not due to age alone, but to other risk factors associated with being a teenage mother. Teenage mothers are more likely than older mothers to be poor and unmarried. They are also shorter, lighter, less educated, and most important — less likely to receive adequate prenatal care.

Young mothers under age seventeen have higher rates of infant mortality than mothers in their twenties and early thirties. Infants born to teenagers are two to three times more likely to be low birthweight than infants born to mothers age 25-29 years and are twice as likely to die before age one.

5   POISONED IN THE WOMB: AN OVERVIEW

FETAL ALCOHOL FACT SHEET

The Children's Trust Foundation

"If women didn't drink anymore during pregnancy, there would never be another baby born with Fetal Alcohol Syndrome or Effect."

Ann Streissguth, Ph.D., University of Washington

WHAT ARE FAS AND FAE?

When mothers drink alcohol while pregnant, their babies could have Fetal Alcohol Syndrome (FAS) or Fetal Alcohol Effect (FAE). FAS and FAE are a group of birth defects that have no cure. People with FAS and FAE have a range of problems as severe as being mentally retarded to less visible problems like difficulty paying attention in school. Maternal use of alcohol might cause a child to:

...be slow or mentally retarded

...have learning problems, with a lower IQ

...look different than other children

...be hyperactive, with a short attention span

...be small for his age

...have many health problems

FACTS

• FAS is the #1 known cause of mental retardation in the

From "A Children's Trust Foundation Fact Sheet", reprinted in the record of a Congressional Hearing before the House Committee on Interior and Insular Affairs, March 5, 1992.

United States, and one of the three leading causes of birth defects.

- Each year over 40,000 American children are born with defects because their mother drank alcohol when pregnant.

- The effects of FAS never go away. People with FAS have the disabilities they are born with, including mental retardation, throughout their lives.

CAN FAS AND FAE BE PREVENTED?

Yes, they are both 100% preventable. When a woman stays away from alcohol (beer, wine, hard liquor and wine coolers) during pregnancy, her baby will not have FAS or FAE.

- Women planning a pregnancy should stop drinking alcohol before trying to conceive and should not drink throughout pregnancy and nursing.

- Women who drink and have an unplanned pregnancy should quit drinking as soon as they suspect they are pregnant.

- Heavy drinkers should avoid pregnancy until they think they can stay away from alcohol for the nine months from conception to birth.

HOW MUCH IS TOO MUCH?

There is no known safe amount of alcohol for a pregnant woman. When a woman drinks, her baby drinks because the alcohol passes directly through the placenta to the baby.

FOR MORE INFORMATION ABOUT...

Alcohol use: call the 24-hour Alcohol/Drug Help Line, 1-800-562-1240.

Birth defects: call March of Dimes, 1-800-345-5188.

FAS diagnosis: call Children's Hospital Medical Center
Fetal Risk Clinic, (206) 526-2208.

This fact sheet: call Children's Trust Foundation, (206) 343-5911.

Financial Contributions:
send to Fetal Alcohol Syndrome Fund, c/o Seattle Foundation, Suite 510, 425 Pike Street, Seattle, WA, 98101.

---

6   POISONED IN THE WOMB: AN OVERVIEW

FETAL ALCOHOL SYNDROME: THE TEN COMMON MISCONCEPTIONS

Ann Pytkowicz Streissguth, Ph.D.

1. FAS means mental retardation.

* *Some people with FAS are mentally retarded; others are not.*
* *People with FAS can have normal intelligence.*
* *People with FAS are brain damaged and have specific areas of strengths and weaknesses. It is similar to people who have sustained brain injury from an auto accident.*

2. The behavior problems associated with FAS/FAE are the result of poor parenting or a bad environment.

* *Being brain damaged can lead to behavior problems because brain damaged people don't process information the same way that other people do, so they don't always behave like others expect them to.*
* *Brain damaged children can be hard to raise in the best environment.*
* *Parents of children with FAS/FAE need help and support, not criticism.*

3. Children with FAS/FAE will outgrow their behavior problems as they mature.

* *Unfortunately, they do not. FAS lasts a lifetime, but the way the individual behaves and the type of problems he/she exhibits can change with age.*
* *It takes a longer period of sheltered living for brain damaged chil-*

dren to "grow up".

4. To admit people with FAS/FAE are brain damaged is to give up on them.

- *Have we given up on children with other birth defects? No!*

- *We need continuing research to understand the needs of patients with FAS and how to help them. We will learn how to help them when we decide to invest money and energy into research on this problem.*

5. Diagnosing people with FAS/FAE will label them for life.

- *A diagnosis tells you what the problem is, helps you figure out how to treat the problem, and relieves the person with FAS/FAE of having to meet unrealistic expectations.*

6. People with FAS/FAE are unmotivated when they don't keep appointments or act in a way that we consider irresponsible.

- *Probably the explanation lies in memory problems, inability to problem-solve effectively, or simply being overwhelmed.*

- *Sometimes people with FAS/FAE misconstrue reality.*

7. One agency alone can solve any or all of the problems associated with people with FAS/FAE.

- *The multiple needs of patients with FAS/FAE require multiple fronts of intervention and intense inter-agency cooperation.*

8. The numerous problems in dealing with the reality of FAS/FAE will be solved with existing knowledge.

- *Ongoing research is desperately needed, and the magnitude of the problem will make it necessary and compelling to do so.*

9. The problem of FAS/FAE will go away.

- *FAS is 100% preventable, but alcohol is so much a part of our culture and so aggressively marketed to those least able to resist, that active prevention activities must continue on all fronts to safeguard our children's future and the future of our people.*

10. Women have an easy choice not to drink during pregnancy, and through callousness or indifference, permanently damage their children.

- *Biologic mothers of children with FAS need help with their alcoholism and/or with birth control.*

- *Pregnancy is an excellent time for alcohol-abusing women to stop drinking, but they need our help.*

WHAT IS EDITORIAL BIAS?

This activity may be used as an individualized study guide for students in libraries and resource centers or as a discussion catalyst in small group and classroom discussions.

The capacity to recognize an author's point of view is an essential reading skill. The skill to read with insight and understanding involves the ability to detect different kinds of opinions or bias. **Sex bias, race bias, ethnocentric bias, political bias,** and **religious bias** are five basic kinds of opinions expressed in editorials and all literature that attempts to persuade. They are briefly defined below.

FIVE KINDS OF EDITORIAL OPINION OR BIAS

Sex Bias — The expression of dislike for and/or feeling of superiority over the opposite sex or a particular sexual minority

Race Bias — The expression of dislike for and/or feeling of superiority over a racial group

Ethnocentric Bias — The expression of a belief that one's own group, race, religion, culture, or nation is superior. Ethnocentric persons judge others by their own standards and values

Political Bias — The expression of political opinions and attitudes about domestic or foreign affairs

Religious Bias — The expression of a religious belief or attitude

Guidelines

1. From the readings in Chapter One, locate five sentences that provide examples of editorial opinion or bias.

2. Write down each of the above sentences and determine what

kind of bias each sentence represents. Is it **sex bias, race bias, ethnocentric bias, political bias** or **religious bias?**

3. Make up one-sentence statements that would be an example of each of the following: **sex bias, race bias, ethnocentric bias, political bias** or **religious bias.**

4. See if you can locate five sentences that are **factual** statements from the readings in Chapter One.

CHAPTER 2

FETAL ALCOHOL SYNDROME: POINTS AND COUNTERPOINTS

FETAL ALCOHOL SYNDROME: POINTS AND COUNTERPOINTS

DEFINING FETAL ALCOHOL SYNDROME (FAS) AND FETAL ALCOHOL EFFECT (FAE)

Gail Stewart Hand

Gail Stewart Hand wrote the following article for the Knight-Ridder News Service.

Points to Consider:

1. Define fetal alcohol syndrome.

2. Summarize behavioral problems of children with FAS.

3. How is the FAS / FAE diagnosis helpful to the patient?

4. How can FAS / FAE be avoided entirely?

Gail Stewart Hand, "When Babies Become Lifelong Victims," **St. Paul Pioneer Press,** March 21, 1993. Reprinted by permission: Tribune Media Services.

WHAT TO STOP

- *Women planning a pregnancy should stop drinking alcohol before trying to conceive and should not drink throughout pregnancy and nursing.*

- *Women who drink and have an unplanned pregnancy should quit drinking as soon as they suspect they are pregnant.*

- *Heavy drinkers should avoid pregnancy until they think they can stay away from alcohol for the time required for conception, birth and nursing.*

GRAND FORKS, N.D.

They don't want you to know their son's name. We'll call him Chad. He lives in eastern North Dakota. He's now 14. Chad was born with fetal alcohol syndrome, although it was diagnosed only about a year ago.

Chad is adopted, which is typical of children with fetal alcohol syndrome. Most of the mothers of fetal alcohol syndrome children are unable to care for them.

As a baby, his adoptive mother says, Chad would be left alone for days while his mother drank in bars. He would stay in the car, sucking on his lower lip to soothe the hurt of hunger. By the time he was 3 1/2, social workers had permanently removed him from his mother's custody, and he had been in five foster homes. The effects of fetal alcohol syndrome make it hard to rear these children. Usually, mothers give up.

It's also not unusual for fetal alcohol syndrome children to be shunted from one foster home to another. The day his adoptive mother took him home, she was handed a report that said he was mean to other children in foster care and would remain silent for hours, staring off into space. His adoptive mother says she was so happy to get Chad that the report didn't sink in.

When he was four, a psychologist examined him and told his adoptive parents that he would come around. Although he had been badly neglected, he would make progress, they were told. " 'He'll be just fine,' he said," his mother remembers ruefully.

In the years since, Chad was seen by a number of specialists, but "no doctor had ever mentioned fetal alcohol syndrome," his adoptive mother said. She came across his condition almost by

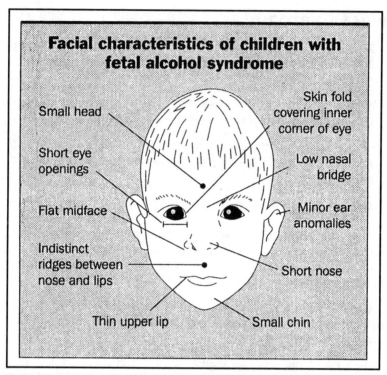

Facial characteristics of children with fetal alcohol syndrome

Small head

Short eye openings

Flat midface

Indistinct ridges between nose and lips

Thin upper lip

Skin fold covering inner corner of eye

Low nasal bridge

Minor ear anomalies

Short nose

Small chin

St. Paul Pioneer Press Graphic, reprinted with permission.

accident, after going to a program on drug abuse.

While other children like to hang around friends, Chad does not. His mother has to make him play. He likes to rake the yard and do other simple, repetitive chores. He doesn't make friends. He can't do regular school work. "You have to drag things out of him," his mother said. "You can't tell how he feels. He masks his emotions." His parents must act as advocates for Chad, telling teachers about fetal alcohol syndrome and what it does to his body and brain. They hope that someday he can make change and tell time.

"I used to tell him he could be anything he wanted to be. He won't be a doctor, won't be the president of the United States," his mother said. Now she has more realistic hopes. "Maybe he could live out of our home."

IF YOU THINK YOUR CHILD HAS FETAL ALCOHOL SYNDROME OR FETAL ALCOHOL EFFECT:

1. Understand the problem

Seek information on the syndrome and determine the alcohol history of your child's biological mother. Discuss your concerns with your family physician and get a diagnosis from an expert on birth defects (a dysmorphologist). You may also need to get help from the biological mother.

2. Find help at school

Find an advocate at the school and discuss placement options for your child. He or she may need an individualized learning plan. Get involved with the school and educate school officials about fetal alcohol syndrome.

3. Utilize community resources

Contact your county social services agencies to determine if they provide any services you and your family can use.

4. Improve relations at home

Maintain consistent structure and supervision in your home. Learn behavior management techniques that will help you avoid crises. Have fun together as a family.

5. Plan for the future

It requires careful planning for a child afflicted with fetal alcohol syndrome to learn to live independently. Encourage your child to learn job skills. Make a long-term financial plan for the child, including disability and medical coverage as needed. Look for supervised living situations as needed.

6. Work to improve community resources

Start or join a community support group.

QUESTIONS & ANSWERS

Q. What is fetal alcohol syndrome?

A. Fetal alcohol syndrome includes brain injury, growth impairment before and after birth, and facial deformities. The syndrome was officially recognized in 1973, as a pattern of mental, physical and behavioral problems. The effects of fetal alcohol syndrome never go away.

Q. What are some of the behavioral problems of children with fetal alcohol syndrome?

A. Impulsiveness, inability to learn from mistakes, lack of discipline and inhibitions. They may be outgoing, loving, trusting. Sometimes, that results in people taking advantage of their gullibility. Children with FAS also have poor memories, decreased attention span, lowered IQ, low achievement, poor judgment and various learning disabilities. As older children, they may drop out of school in frustration and may end up in trouble with the law because of their poor judgment.

Q. How prevalent is fetal alcohol syndrome?

A. Fetal alcohol syndrome is the No. 1 cause of mental retardation in the United States and one of the three leading causes of birth defects. Each year, more than 40,000 American children are born with defects because their mother drank alcohol while pregnant.

Q. If a parent has FAS, does that mean his or her children also will have it?

A. Parents with fetal alcohol syndrome produce normal babies as long as they abstain from alcohol during pregnancy. But their parenting needs lots of support. For example, they will forget to dress a child warmly enough.

Q. When can pregnant women safely drink alcohol?

A. Never. The human brain starts to develop after conception and continues beyond birth. Alcohol kills brain cells. If the pregnant woman drinks in the first trimester, the baby is more likely to have physical malformation, while in the third trimester, there may be behavioral, social and learning problems without physical clues.

Q. How much can a mother drink before damage is done?

A. No one knows what amount of drinking is likely to produce a child with fetal alcohol syndrome. How much harm the alcohol causes depends on such factors as the mother's diet, her overall health and genetic makeup and the age at which she started drinking. In addition, effects vary among embryos.

44

8   FETAL ALCOHOL SYNDROME: POINTS AND COUNTERPOINTS

FAS: A NATIONAL CRISIS

Robin A. LaDue & Barbara A. VonFeldt

Robin A. LaDue, Ph.D., is a Clinical Psychologist. Barbara A. VonFeldt is an Information Specialist at the Department of Psychiatry and Behavioral Sciences at the University of Washington School of Medicine.

Points to Consider:

1. Compare the incidence of FAS nationwide with that found in the Native American community.

2. Explain the significance: "Those [FAS] children are not born into a vacuum."

3. Why should Native American education and prevention efforts be aimed at the school-aged population?

4. Summarize recommended treatment programs.

Excerpted from congressional testimony by Robin A. LaDue and Barbara A. VonFeldt before the House Committee on Interior and Insular Affairs, March 5, 1992.

"If every pregnant woman from this day forward would choose not to drink alcohol during her pregnancy, we would never have another FAS child."

It has now been almost twenty years since the Fetal Alcohol Syndrome (FAS) was first identified by the University of Washington research group. Since that time, several thousand articles have been published documenting that it is, indeed, alcohol consumed prenatally that causes the growth deficiencies, facial and other physical anomalies, and the central nervous system damage that are the markers of FAS. These effects are permanent and have life-long implications for people with FAS or Fetal Alcohol Effect (FAE).

FAS and FAE are believed by some researchers to be the leading known cause of mental retardation in this country. This is a double tragedy as FAS and FAE are totally preventable, the only birth defect that can be completely eradicated. Prevalence figures for FAS run between 1 in 600 to 1 in 750 births, depending upon the drinking pattern of women in a specific community. The number of people impacted by FAE is higher at approximately 1 in 300 to 1 in 350 births. Estimates of the prevalence rate for FAS in Native American country range from those quoted above to as high as 1 in 99 births. However, one of the significant problems facing Indian communities is the lack of adequate studies and data documenting the actual numbers of people with FAS and in what age range these numbers might be concentrated. The latter information is critical in formulating appropriate prevention and treatment programs.

Studies published in the last ten years have shown an increase in the number of Native American women drinking with a recent study estimating that 40% meet the criteria for alcohol dependency. If these studies are accurate, Native American communities are facing an epidemic of children born with life-long, debilitating effects from prenatal alcohol exposure. It is for this reason that the passage of the proposed legislation is so critical.

LONG-TERM EFFECTS OF PRENATAL ALCOHOL EXPOSURE

FAS is characterized by a distinct, consistent pattern of prenatal growth deficiency in three parameters — height, weight, and head

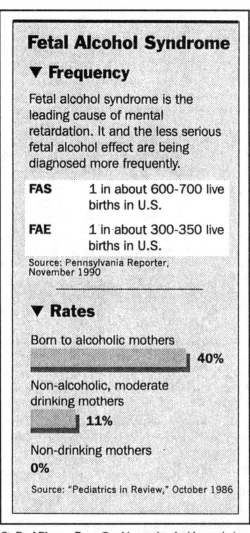

Fetal Alcohol Syndrome

▼ Frequency

Fetal alcohol syndrome is the leading cause of mental retardation. It and the less serious fetal alcohol effect are being diagnosed more frequently.

FAS	1 in about 600-700 live births in U.S.
FAE	1 in about 300-350 live births in U.S.

Source: Pennsylvania Reporter, November 1990

▼ Rates

Born to alcoholic mothers
40%

Non-alcoholic, moderate drinking mothers
11%

Non-drinking mothers
0%

Source: "Pediatrics in Review," October 1986

St. Paul Pioneer Press Graphic, reprinted with permission.

circumference; facial anomalies; and central nervous system (CNS) damage. The central nervous system damage is pervasive and occurs even in the absence of marked growth deficiencies and facial abnormalities. The psychosocial, behavioral, and cognitive problems facing patients and their families with FAS and FAE include delays in walking, talking and toilet training, difficulties in following directions, distractibility, and hyperactivity.

Other signs are memory deficits, poor comprehension of social rules and expectations, low self-esteem, depression, social and sexual exploitation, suicidal ideation and attempts, and other psychiatric disorders. The cause of these problems, brain damage from prenatal alcohol exposure, is permanent and actually increases in severity as the person gets older. It is for these reasons that prevention of FAS is so important. Once the child is born, there is no repairing the brain; the damage is there for good.

It is also important when discussing the long-term consequences of prenatal alcohol use to remember the families of patients born with FAS and FAE. These children are not born into a vacuum. One of the more sobering findings from a longitudinal study carried out by the University of Washington Fetal Alcohol and Drug Unit was the fact that over half of the mothers of children in the study were dead by the time the child was 16 years old. A significant portion of these women died by the time the child was five. The devastation of families by alcohol meant that many of the children diagnosed with FAS or FAE have been neglected, sexually and physically abused, and moved from home to home, often before the age of five.

In Native American communities, these issues become even more acute if there are not sober foster homes for these children to be raised in nor prevention and treatment programs available to help provide support and treatment for alcohol abuse. These people have, all too often, been an underserved population; this is true in terms of both alcohol programs and programs designed to meet the needs of people with FAS and their families.

RECOMMENDATIONS

The primary goal of those working in the field of alcohol-related birth defects is the total eradication of FAS and FAE; to this end, it is crucial that culturally appropriate and community specific prevention programs be designed and implemented. Such programs would include the use of traditional Native strengths such as the extended family and traditional healers.

Successful examples of community actions and programs include the efforts made by the Alkili Lake Band and the Indian Aunt program instituted by the Lummi Tribe of Washington State. The Indian Health Service now has a program out of Albuquerque designed to help Native communities increase awareness of FAS. It is also important that tribal councils educate themselves regarding FAS and that a mandatory two years sobriety be a requirement

FETAL ALCOHOL SYNDROME AND FETAL ALCOHOL EFFECT

Fetal alcohol syndrome (FAS) is a medical condition characterized by physical and behavioral disabilities resulting from heavy exposure to alcohol before birth. A child with a history of prenatal alcohol exposure but not all the physical or behavioral symptoms of FAS may be categorized as having fetal alcohol effect (FAE) or alcohol related birth defects (ARBD). It should be noted that FAE is not the less severe form of FAS: rather, a child with FAE does not have all the physical abnormalities of FAS.

Early Childhood Project, School of Medicine, South Dakota University in a report titled **Fetal Alcohol Syndrome**, 1992

for anyone wishing to serve on a tribal council. The sobriety requirement would also apply to anyone employed in teaching, social services, and the health care system on reservations and in Native communities. Physicians, nurses, teachers, and social service personnel should be required to have continuing education in the field of alcohol-related birth defects.

Other education and prevention efforts should be aimed at the Native American youth. Many of these children begin to drink before the age of 12. Native teenage girls have a pregnancy rate twice that of the rest of the United States. Given these two facts, prevention efforts need to start in grade school and continue through high school. Specific curricula aimed at Native youngsters need to be developed and disseminated. Community-specific warning signs, posters, and brochures should be placed in doctor's offices, tribal offices, and social services offices where they can be seen by community members.

TREATMENT

While these suggestions address the issue of prevention, treatment concerns are pressing for all social and ethnic groups in America. As indicated, the problems experienced by patients with FAS and their families increase in severity the older the patient becomes. The hyperactivity, and memory and social deficits noted in young children lead to school problems, employment difficulties, and social problems including criminal behavior and incarceration, sexual exploitation, and drug and alcohol problems. Of the patients with FAS and FAE that have been followed, only a very small percentage are able to meet their own financial, residential, and personal needs.

Therefore, treatment programs need to include special education and vocational training components that emphasize skills leading to the patient functioning in society in the least restrictive, but safest possible environment. Classroom programs that focus on such skills, coupled with long-term care, including adult residential care, are desperately needed. Respite care for families, medical care for FAS patients past the age of 18, financial support and guardianship, are also areas that require funding.

CONCLUSION

In summation, the passage of the Comprehensive Indian Fetal Alcohol Syndrome Prevention and Treatment Act would be a significant step in addressing the following four areas:

1. Prevention is always more cost efficient than treatment. According to former Senator John Binkley, in an Alaska State Legislature report, the conservative estimate of costs related to providing services to one person born with FAS across his lifespan is $1.4 million dollars. If this figure is multiplied by the estimated 41,000 children born every year with alcohol-related birth defects, it is staggering. If the monies spent for the services needed by just one child were put towards prevention, the long-term savings are incalculable.

2. This Act is a chance to acknowledge the needs of America's first citizens and to provide a chance for the next generation of Native American children.

3. Passage of the Act will provide information and services to children. The proposed legislation will help send a message to Native American children that they are valuable and that their potential is too important to simply throw away.

4. Children, adults, and families affected by FAS have only those who are willing to speak out on this subject and, more importantly, those who are willing to listen. Passage of this Act signifies a willingness to listen to those of "The Broken Cord", to those who cannot speak for themselves, to those who are forever outside the circle of society. Passage of this Act is an acknowledgement that, there but for the grace of God, go any of us.

9   FETAL ALCOHOL SYNDROME: POINTS AND COUNTERPOINTS

MISDIRECTED CRUSADE

Stanton Peele

Stanton Peele is a psychologist and health researcher at Mathematical Policy Research Institute, Princeton University. He is the author of Diseasing of America: Addiction Treatment Out of Control.

Points to Consider:

1. How does the author describe the book by Michael Dorris called *The Broken Cord*?

2. Describe the reasons for the author's belief that the dangers of fetal alcohol syndrome (FAS) and fetal alcohol effect (FAE) have been greatly exaggerated.

3. Who is Ralph Hingson and what did his study show?

4. Why has the crusade against drinking during pregnancy been misdirected?

5. Is any level of drinking safe during pregnancy?

Reprinted with permission from the July 1990 issue of **Reason** Magazine. Copyright 1990 by the Reason Foundation, 2716 Ocean Park Blvd., Suite 1062, Santa Monica, CA 90405.

The women most likely to give birth to damaged babies are not affected by messages tailored to the middle class.

A growing number of pregnant women in the United States avoid alcohol as if it were thalidomide. The pronouncements of government officials, journalists, and other professional alarmists have convinced them that drinking any amount of alcohol during pregnancy endangers the fetus. This new conventional wisdom is embodied in the federal warning that now appears on every bottle of wine, beer, and liquor manufactured for sale in this country: "According to the Surgeon General, women should not drink alcoholic beverages during pregnancy because of the risk of birth defects."

CAMPAIGNS

The horrible effects of fetal alcohol syndrome — which include mental retardation, cardiac defects, and facial deformities — were publicized throughout the 1980s. More recently, *The Broken Cord*, Michael Dorris's account of his experiences in raising an adopted Native American child suffering from FAS, has renewed the storm of anxiety about alcohol consumption during pregnancy. Dorris's book warns people that the danger of drinking by pregnant women has been vastly underestimated. The news media has been eager to amplify that view.

The success of the campaign against drinking during pregnancy demonstrates that any attacks on alcohol, no matter how far-fetched, misleading, or counter-productive, are nowadays immune from criticism. By blurring important distinctions, reports on FAS have generated needless worry among occasional or moderate drinkers while distracting attention from the real problems of prenatal care.

RESEARCH

People have long recognized that heavy alcohol consumption is a risky behavior for pregnant women. But U.S. researchers first used the term fetal alcohol syndrome in the early 1970s to describe severe abnormalities in the newborn children of alcoholic mothers, including brain damage and readily observable physical deformities.

Such children are quite rare, however, even among heavy

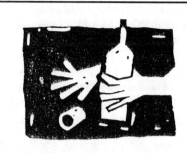

drinkers. In their 1984 book *Alcohol and the Fetus*, based on a comprehensive survey of the research, Dr. Henry Rosett and Lyn Weiner of Boston University reported that studies find FAS occurs in only 2 percent to 10 percent of children born to alcohol abusers. Furthermore, they reported that in every one of the 400 FAS cases described in the scientific literature, the mother "was a chronic alcoholic who drank heavily during pregnancy."

The infrequency of FAS has prompted researchers to expand their focus beyond the severe birth defects sometimes caused by heavy drinking. Hence "fetal alcohol effect", which refers to more subtle impairment that might ordinarily escape attention. Closely tied to the rather vague notion of fetal alcohol effect is the suggestion that light or moderate drinking might also be dangerous. Warnings about FAS, fetal alcohol effect, and the alleged risks of any drinking during pregnancy get tossed together in the news media.

An article by Dr. Elisabeth Rosenthal in *The New York Times Magazine*, "When a Pregnant Woman Drinks," begins with a horrific tale of an FAS victim. In this case, not only did the eight-year-old girl have FAS, but so did her siblings and her mother. Immediately following this extreme example, the article describes how Dr. Claire Coles, as FAS expert, has begun to "see the survivors of drinking pregnancies everywhere." For example, upon visiting a reform school, Coles observed, "My God, half these kids look alcohol-affected."

FALSE IMPRESSIONS

The bait-and-switch juxtaposition of Coles's observation with the severe FAS case creates the false impression that such alcohol-related birth defects are common. Alcohol-affected, the term used by Coles, is generally applied to infants who have problems that fall short of FAS, such as irritability, attention deficits, hyperactivity, or developmental delays. The condition cannot be discerned simply by looking at a child. But for those who see fetal alcohol effect "everywhere", even criminal behavior may be the result of a mother's drinking. (Attorneys representing condemned California murderer Robert Alton Harris offered such an argument.)

Increasingly, problems such as delinquency and learning disabilities are being attributed to maternal drinking. Combined with warnings about moderate alcohol consumption, this tendency is likely to cause irrational guilt among many parents. The mother of a child who gets into trouble or has difficulty in school will start to wonder if this has anything to do with the wine she occasionally drank during her pregnancy.

Weiner, co-author of *Alcohol and the Fetus*, has described the anxiety caused by exaggeration of the danger from drinking during pregnancy: "Women are worrying about wine vinegar in their salad dressing and getting hysterical about the risk of eating rum cake, and they think they need an abortion after they hear the scare stories."

What grounds, if any, are there for such alarm? Rosenthal's article is accompanied by a subhead that warns, "New Studies Show That Even Moderate Consumption Can Be Harmful to the Unborn Child." But the article cites only one study to support this claim: In 1988, a University of Pittsburgh researcher found "minor anomalies" in children of mothers who consumed less than one drink a day during pregnancy.

Rosenthal has latched onto one highly unusual finding in a sea of contradictory evidence, ignoring a host of studies that have found no effect from consumption of two drinks or less a day. In 1984, Rosett and Weiner concluded, "the recommendation that all women should abstain from drinking during pregnancy is not based on scientific evidence." The overwhelming majority of studies since then have also failed to find evidence that moderate drinking harms the fetus. In fact, Dr. Jack Mendelson, a distinguished alcohol researcher at Harvard Medical School, has declared, "It is possible that some doses of alcohol, low or moderate, may improve the probability for healthy pregnancies and healthy offspring."

LACK OF EVIDENCE

Given the rush to condemn any drinking during pregnancy despite the lack of research evidence to support such a policy, you might guess that fetal alcohol effect, if not FAS itself, is a widespread phenomenon. But the Centers for Disease Control estimate that 8,000 "alcohol-damaged babies" are born each year, which works out to a rate of 2.7 for every 1,000 live births (0.27%).

Yet *New York Times* health columnist Jane Brody offered a much higher figure in 1986, when she announced, "An estimated 50,000 babies born last year suffered from prenatal alcohol exposure." (Brody, by the way, does not think it's enough merely to abstain from alcohol during pregnancy: "Even drinking before pregnancy [as little as one drink a day] may have a negative result," she reported.)

Rosenthal does not offer her own estimate, but she says the CDC figure seems low, apparently because "on some Indian reservations, 25 percent of all children are reportedly afflicted." But as she later notes, "The CDC data show that the syndrome is 30 times more commonly reported in Native Americans than it is in whites, and six times more common in blacks." These figures indicate that alcohol-related damage among babies of white, middle-class women is actually less common than 2.7 cases per 1,000, since all groups are averaged together in producing the overall rate.

MIDDLE-CLASS WOMEN

Indeed, it's not clear what the middle-class women who read the *Times* can learn from the experience of grossly dysfunctional families such as the one described at the beginning of Rosenthal's article or from reports about Native American children such as the mentally retarded in *The Broken Cord.* For one thing, styles of drinking vary widely across racial and socioeconomic groups.

White, middle-class women are more likely to drink than black women (and low-income women generally), but they tend to drink moderately. Black women are more likely to abstain, but those who don't are more likely to drink heavily. The fact that FAS rates are much higher among low-income minorities therefore contradicts the hypothesis that moderate drinking during pregnancy is damaging and that higher rates of abstinence would reduce FAS.

And a 1982 study by Boston University researcher Ralph Hingson suggests that other factors in the lives of poor, ghetto-dwelling women contribute to birth defects that have been ascribed solely to alcohol. After studying a sample of 1,700 women in Boston City Hospital, Hingson concluded that "neither level of drinking prior to pregnancy nor during pregnancy was significantly related to infant growth measures, congenital abnormality, or [other] features compatible with fetal alcohol syndrome."

MISDIRECTED CRUSADE

Rather, a combination of factors — including smoking, malnutrition, and poor health care — seems to be responsible for low birth weight and other problems often attributed to drinking. "The results underline the difficulty in isolating and proclaiming single factors as the cause of abnormal fetal development," Hingson and his colleagues wrote.

So the crusade against drinking during pregnancy is misdirected in several ways. It focuses on moderate rather than heavy drinking, on middle-class rather than low-income mothers, and on alcohol consumption rather than the set of behaviors that increases the risk of birth defects. The women most likely to give birth to damaged babies — the ones who abuse alcohol and drugs, smoke, and neglect their health — are not affected by messages tailored to the middle class.

The error in strategy is especially troubling given the nation's relatively poor performance in prenatal care. The number of birth defects in the United States has doubled in the last 25 years. While the U.S. neonatal death rate dropped in the 1980s, it still compares unfavorably with those of European nations, Japan, Australia, Singapore, Bermuda, and even Guam. Shrill warnings about low levels of drinking during pregnancy may make health experts feel virtuous, but they won't improve those figures one bit. Developing comprehensive community programs for high-risk mothers would help, but this requires more than Sunday-supplement alarmism.

10   FETAL ALCOHOL SYNDROME: POINTS AND COUNTERPOINTS

DISASTER ON THE RESERVATION

Tom Daschle & Ben Nighthorse Campbell

Tom Daschle wrote the following comments while serving as a Democratic Senator from South Dakota. Ben Nighthorse Campbell wrote the following comments while serving as a Democratic Congressman from the State of Colorado.

Points to Consider:

1. What is the estimated cost of services for one person with FAS?

2. Summarize the provisions of the Comprehensive Fetal Alcohol Syndrome Prevention and Treatment Act.

3. How might drinking during pregnancy be regarded as child abuse?

4. Cite evidence that United States treatment programs are inadequate.

Excerpted from testimony by Tom Daschle and Ben Nighthorse Campbell before the House Committee on Interior and Insular Affairs, March 5, 1992.

This is not a disease that needs to be cured, but one that can, and must be 100 percent prevented.

Representative Ben Nighthorse Campbell's remarks follow:

Fetal Alcohol Syndrome, known as FAS, is a devastating disease that affects the children of mothers who drink alcohol during pregnancy. These children have a wide range of problems from hyperactivity and reduced IQ scores to organ dysfunction and life threatening seizures. Fetal Alcohol Effect, FAE, is a disorder related to FAS but the symptoms are less severe.

Approximately one in 500 children born in the United States today are born with Fetal Alcohol Syndrome. The number for Fetal Alcohol Effect is one in 300. These numbers make FAS the leading cause of mental retardation at birth in this country. This fact is particularly discouraging because FAS is the only birth defect identified that is 100 percent preventable.

INDIAN COUNTRY

In Indian country, incidence of FAS and FAE is much higher. Approximately one in 99 American Indians are born with FAS. This means one in 99 Indian children will be denied the opportunity to learn and grow as they should. They will be denied the opportunity to live their lives with healthy bodies and independent spirits, and this nation will be denied their contributions to society.

I'm sorry to report that the devastating effects of Fetal Alcohol Syndrome is more pervasive in some communities than others. I will not be the only person at this hearing to point to studies that find one in four children born on the Pine Ridge and Rosebud Reservations have Fetal Alcohol Syndrome. These innocent children will never have the opportunities of a healthy mind and body that most of us take for granted. Their communities are losing much of the creativity and ideas of a quarter of their people.

THE COST

Those with FAS are far more likely to have drug and alcohol problems as adults. These children seem to be struck with a reduced ability to reason. They have difficulties understanding that one event or action can lead directly to a consequential event or situation. Ultimately, this causes adults with FAS to be much more likely to produce FAS children themselves.

The costs of Fetal Alcohol Syndrome to society are staggering. A report from the Alaska State Legislature estimated that the cost of services and lost productivity from one person with FAS is approximately $1.4 million dollars. In spite of all of this bad news, there is hope for ending the tragedy of FAS. Dr. Ann Streissguth, a leader in FAS research, has simplified this issue for us. She said, "If every pregnant woman from this day forward would choose not to drink alcohol during her pregnancy, we would never have another FAS child."

The science is simple. If mothers do not drink alcohol, any alcohol, during the nine months of their pregnancy, they will not give birth to a child with Fetal Alcohol Syndrome. We know how to put an end to FAS. This is not a disease that needs to be cured, but one that can, and must be 100 percent prevented.

SOCIAL PROBLEMS

Our job is to address the social and educational problems that create an environment where expecting mothers abuse alcohol. We must educate women about the dangers of alcohol consumption during pregnancy, and assist those who may have difficulty curbing their consumption during critical fetal development.

My bill, The Comprehensive Indian Fetal Alcohol Syndrome Prevention and Treatment Act, begins to address these problems. It authorizes the Secretary of Health and Human Services to make grants for community training education and prevention programs for FAS and FAE. It would provide alcohol and substance abuse treatment to high-risk women and would provide support services, advocacy and information to FAS afflicted persons.

This legislation is only the first step in eliminating FAS in Indian communities and throughout the nation. I am pleased that this issue has received so much attention and that many of my colleagues are also studying and proposing programs to eliminate FAS. I look forward to working with Chairman Miller and other Members of this Committee and Congress to prevent and eliminate the wastefulness of Fetal Alcohol Syndrome.

When the baby started to cry, the smell of cheap wine was on her breath.

Senator Tom Daschle's remarks follow:

I particularly want to highlight my colleague Congressman Ben Nighthorse Campbell's prominent role in the effort to address this tragedy. He has worked long and tirelessly to heighten public and Congressional awareness of this issue, and I am pleased and honored to be working side-by-side with him to develop real solutions to a very real problem.

I became interested in — and concerned about — Fetal Alcohol Syndrome when I held a hearing in 1990 on Indian child abuse on the Rosebud Sioux Reservation in my own State of South Dakota. In the hundreds of hearings in which I have participated, never have I been so moved or so shaken as by the testimony I heard that day. One of the witnesses, Jeanean Grey Eagle, told a story about an incident on Pine Ridge which graphically illustrates the problem of FAS on that reservation:

"A woman came to the hospital ready to deliver. She had never been in a prenatal clinic before. This woman was obviously intoxicated. When the baby was born — a little girl — she had difficulty breathing and was taken to another room for medical care. When the baby started to cry, the smell of cheap wine was on her breath. It was very strong. This baby would not breathe because she was technically passed out! This is child abuse."

CHILD ABUSE

In fact, prenatal child abuse by a mother who drinks while pregnant may be one of the most prevalent forms of child abuse in our nation. Unfortunately, this kind of abuse can permanently and irreparably impair the fetus. It may lead to the birth of a retarded child with facial malformations, painful seizures, and lifelong impairment of learning and social functions.

Fetal Alcohol Syndrome is one of the leading causes of mental retardation and birth defects in the world. The child born with FAS is highly likely to become addicted to drugs or alcohol, break the law, cost society millions of dollars in medical, social, and rehabilitative costs — and perhaps most tragically, bear another FAS child.

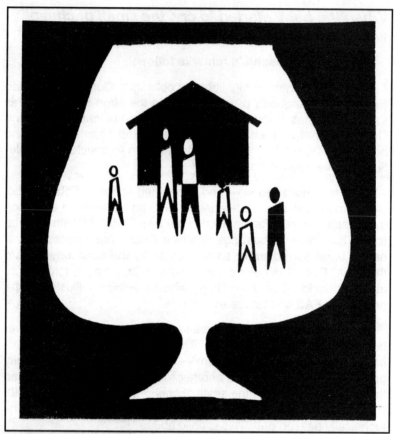

Engage / Social Action

The National Institute on Alcohol Abuse and Alcoholism estimates that one out of every six women of childbearing age may drink enough to threaten her unborn baby.

While FAS cuts across all races, nationalities, social and economic boundaries, there are few places where its effects are so devastating as among Native Americans. The Indian Health Service estimates that the rate of FAS among Indians is 30 times the rate among whites. Studies have indicated that one in four children at Pine Ridge and other reservations are born to mothers who drink while pregnant. As a result, the infant mortality rate on this reservation is worse than that of many countries such as Cuba, Bulgaria, and Peru.

ALASKA NATIVE HEALTH SERVICE

For many years, Fetal Alcohol Syndrome and Fetal Alcohol Effect were kept well hidden. The idea that women were somehow contributing to such an unhealthy pregnancy outcome was unconscionable. Fetal Alcohol Syndrome did not even have a name until 1973. Less than 20 years later, alcohol-related birth defects had become the leading cause of mental retardation in the U.S. FAS occurs far more frequently among our Native population than in the general population.

Anne M. Walker, Executive Director of Alaska Native Health Board in testimony before the **House Interior and Insular Affairs Committee**, March 5, 1992

SOLUTIONS

There is one ray of hope for this problem: unlike so many matters with which we deal in Congress for which the solutions are either unknown or the problem intractable, this is a problem whose solution is clear. FAS is 100% preventable. What we lack is not the definition of the problem nor an understanding of the solution. What we lack is the commitment. Here are a few examples of our inadequate response:

• The publicly funded treatment system in the United States is only able to serve 11% of the more than 280,000 pregnant alcohol- and drug-dependent women who seek treatment.

• Two-thirds of the hospitals surveyed by the House Select Committee on Children reported they had no place to which to refer their pregnant addicts.

• In New York City, a survey of treatment programs found that pregnant addicted women were refused service by more than half of all the available programs.

To deal with Fetal Alcohol Syndrome, we must have a vigorous public awareness campaign targeted at pregnant women; better prevention and treatment programs for alcoholic women; additional research on the prevalence of, and best treatment for, FAS; better medical and social services for FAS children; and better criteria for diagnosing FAS.

NATIVE AMERICANS

Nowhere is this need more pressing than among Native Americans. The legislation which Rep. Campbell has proposed is a very concrete and important beginning to deal with this national tragedy. This bill would make grants to tribes to establish FAS programs for training, education, and prevention programs, and would provide treatment to high risk women. It will go a long way toward addressing FAS among Native Americans.

In the Senate, I have introduced a bill which would allow states the option of providing comprehensive residential treatment programs under Medicaid. It has a specific provision to increase services to Native Americans. That bill is under consideration by the Committee on Finance, and I have every expectation that it will be favorably acted on. Along with Reps. Campbell, Richardson, and Synar, Senator Bingaman and I are drafting new legislation which will markedly increase the research, education, prevention, and treatment programs which are so essential if we are to put an end to this tragedy.

11   FETAL ALCOHOL SYNDROME: POINTS AND COUNTERPOINTS

THE SITUATION IS IMPROVING

Cecelia Firethunder

Cecelia Firethunder is an enrolled member of the Oglala Sioux Tribe, Pine Ridge, South Dakota. Firethunder serves as the tribe's Health Planner. Her comments are made in response to House of Representatives Report 1332 entitled "Comprehensive Indian Alcohol Syndrome Prevention and Treatment Act".

Points to Consider:

1. Describe the makeup and purpose of the Pine Ridge community FAS group.

2. What efforts need to be coordinated by a successful community FAS program?

3. Explain the consensus that "all major health problems affecting Indian women are based on psychosocial factors."

4. What is "women-specific" treatment for alcoholism?

Excerpted from testimony by Cecelia Firethunder before the House Committee on Interior and Insular Affairs, March 5, 1992.

*But they have been making some wonderful head-
way in addressing issues around alcohol abuse.*

The Pine Ridge Reservation is home to approximately 22,000 Lakotas who live on 4,500 square miles of land. They are considered the poorest, unhealthiest, highest unemployed, and the highest risk for many other problems. But they have been making some wonderful headway in addressing issues around alcohol abuse. Especially on FAS/FAE, despite all the negatives, there is a strong sense of community with a high awareness of the incidence of FAS/FAE on the reservations. Along with this awareness have been some training for Headstart, health care providers, community organizations and the development of a reservation-wide work group to look at FAS/FAE.

THE COMMUNITY

This group of community people represent most of the agencies, school, federal programs, state programs, tribal programs and parents. The purpose of this group was to get a sense of: What was happening? What was working? Who was doing what? and What needs to happen?

The group brought to the gatherings much information and resources with many having attended some training on FAS/FAE. As the group began working on the needs of the community, the task became overwhelming as our community was very large with many institutions and agencies to negotiate with. The time it would take to put together an FAS/FAE Program could not be found as most of the group were employed full-time in their jobs.

We attempted to continue with the planning and meetings but we realized we needed a fully funded office and staff to coordinate all the agencies and entities, to put together and implement a plan from prevention to the long-term care of FAS/FAE individuals, training for community, families and caretakers and educating these children.

TRIBAL COMMUNITIES' RESPONSE TO FAS/FAE

1. Each tribe or urban community should set up an FAS Program to coordinate education, prevention, intervention, diagnostic, and treatment efforts across all community agencies.

2. FAS/FAE awareness and education materials should be "trib-

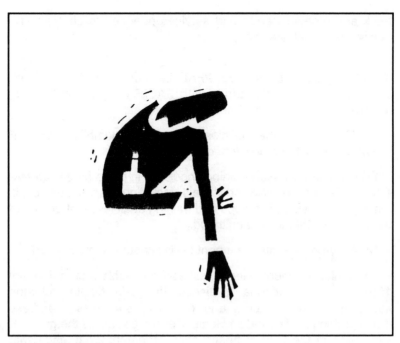

Engage / Social Action

al specific" to meet needs of all age groups. Special emphasis for child-bearing age (male/female), considered high-risk.

3. FAS awareness and inservice programs should be ongoing for all community agencies, schools and those involved with FAS/FAE individuals and families.

4. Pre-natal screening programs should be developed at each service unit, clinic and health center to identify high-risk women.

5. Screening programs should be developed to be used in pediatric clinics, Headstart, Early Childhood Components and schools.

6. School boards and schools should develop special education programs specifically for FAS/FAE children. Teachers should be specially trained to work with these children. All teachers should be trained to assess/screen students.

7. Each tribe and urban community should develop a committee to assess the incidence of FAS/FAE within its community/population for all ages, and develop a plan to meet needs of all affected.

8. An FAS registry should be set up by each tribal community to

track and monitor needs and services provided to children and families over their lifetime.

9. Tribal courts and legal system should develop processes for addressing legal issues on FAS/FAE, i.e., court ordered treatment, advocates for children/adults with FAS/FAE to protect rights, maternal rights, adoptions, and foster care, etc.

10. Community/tribal policies from birth to death of FAS/FAE individuals should be developed.

11. Community based training should be in place for all caretakers and families of FAS individuals, including respite care, crisis management, support groups and training at all levels of growth of the child from infancy to adulthood.

12. A woman-specific treatment facility should be maintained.

The Indian Womens' Health Issues Roundtable met in January 1991 in Tucson, Arizona, to discuss the major health problems facing Indian women today and to develop strategies to address these problems. The Indian Health Service convened the group of experts from the field of health care, research, tribal leadership and community development to develop consensus around major health problems.

It was the consensus of the Indian Womens' Health Roundtable that virtually all the major health problems affecting Indian women are based on psychosocial factors. Poverty, racism, sexism, abuse and cultural bias are all contributing factors to the prevention, intervention, early detection and treatment of such major killers as cervical cancer, type 11 diabetes, cirrhosis of the liver and violence. If the Indian Health Service and tribal communities are to effectively address Indian womens' health, they must understand her relationship to her cultural, social, physical and spiritual environment.

ROUNDTABLE RECOMMENDATIONS:

Participants felt strongly that alcoholism and its multi-generational effect is the root of most health problems experienced by Indian women. Providing treatment for addiction was not enough. Attention must be paid to the cultural and social experiences of Indian women, while in the treatment setting. Ideally, women-specific treatment should be made available in all areas of health for Indian women, to get at the basic question, "What is the pain I am trying to numb?" The link between child abuse, child sexual abuse and early childhood trauma and later substance abuse cannot be ignored for the female population, and should be integrated into the continuum of recovery.

SPECIFIC RECOMMENDATIONS

• "Treatment" programs should be renamed as "Healing Centers" to promote wholeness, to be culturally sensitive, to bring the community into the process and to reduce isolation.

• Healing programs specifically addressing the unique needs of Indian women should be promoted and funded. There should be at least one woman-specific treatment program in each Indian Health Service (IHS) area.

• Research, education, prevention and services related to FAS/FAE should be promoted and funded by IHS, including assessment and treatment. Substance abuse treatment for pregnant women must be considered a priority in developing new treatment centers.

• A national conference on Indian Women and Substance Abuse should be planned to focus attention on the unique needs of Indian women, to showcase successful programs, to share ideas, to stimulate research and to empower Indian women to begin to heal themselves.

• IHS should convene a national "think tank" to address issues of pregnant abusers, legal issues, ethical issues, treatment issues and to assist tribal leadership to respond to the problem.

• Support groups should be encouraged and reinforced in Indian communities, such as Talking Circles, Womens' Groups, Mens' Groups, Teen Groups, Aftercare Groups, and Survivors' Groups. These groups should be supported financially and politically.

12   FETAL ALCOHOL SYNDROME: POINTS AND COUNTERPOINTS

FAS AMONG NORTH AMERICAN INDIANS: OVERVIEW OF SCIENTIFIC LITERATURE

Philip A. May

Philip A. May, Ph.D., is the Director of the Center on Alcoholism, Substance Abuse and Addictions at the University of New Mexico. The Center is located at 2350 Alamo, S.E., Albuquerque, New Mexico 87106.

Points to Consider:

1. What general patterns emerge among Indian women who produce FAS/FAE children?

2. Compare the incidence of FAS in the various ethnic groups of the United States.

3. What are the general characteristics of successful FAS prevention programs?

4. What does the author believe to be the most effective makeup of an ARBD prevention group?

Excerpted from testimony by Philip A. May before the House Committee on Interior and Insular Affairs, March 5, 1992.

1. The scientifically reliable and complete epidemiologic research on Alcohol-Related Birth Defects (ARBD) among Indians is limited to a few studies in the published literature.

2. This literature examines the prevalence of the most severe forms of ARBD as they are manifest in Indian populations. These severe forms are Fetal Alcohol Syndrome (FAS) and Fetal Alcohol Effect (FAE) both of which are produced by the more abusive and chronic drinking women. These two levels of damage are clinically quite diagnosable from various physical anomalies and a history of maternal alcohol consumption.

3. Lower levels of ARBD damage have been consistently found in laboratory studies of animals,[14] but are currently difficult to impossible to diagnose in any human populations.

4. The existing, published studies on North American Indians show the following patterns:

• The rates of FAS and FAE vary widely over time and by American Indian community. Some Indian communities have rates comparable to U.S. averages, while others are higher.

• FAS and FAE appear with higher frequency among Plains culture tribes than among some other cultural groups of Indians.[9]

• Generally, a mother who produces one FAS or FAE child may well have one or more subsequent children who are affected. The average range is from 1.3 to 1.6 damaged children per mother. A few mothers have had up to five FAS and FAE children.[9, 11]

• The mothers who produce the most severely damaged children (FAS and FAE) are quite concentrated within most Indian populations. These mothers make up between 3.9 to 33.3 per 1,000 of the women of childbearing age (15-44 years of age).[9]

• Mothers who produce FAS and FAE children are frequently living very chaotic lifestyles within alcohol abusing peer clusters. Because of this lifestyle, over 70% of Indian children with FAS and FAE are in foster or adoptive placement by the time they are several years old, and a high percentage of the mothers wind up dead from alcohol-related causes within a decade after the birth of the first FAS and FAE child.[9, 12, 13]

5. The prevalence of FAS and FAE in Indian communities as established in the scientific literature can briefly be summarized as follows:

• In the Southwestern U.S. the retrospective rates of FAS and FAE for children born in 1968-1982 were found to be:[9]

2.2 per 1,000 children for the Navajo

2.4 per 1,000 children for the Pueblo

17.9 per 1,000 children for the Southwestern Plains tribes

• However, in the same Southwestern U.S. study, children born from 1978-1982 had higher FAS and FAE rates, probably indicating a rise in the problem:[9]

5.2 per 1,000 children for the Navajo

5.7 per 1,000 children for the Pueblo

17.5 per 1,000 children for the Southwestern Plains tribes

• In northern Canada, Asante et al[2] found FAS and FAE to affect 46 per 1,000 Native children in the Yukon and 25 per 1,000 in northern British Columbia.

• In a very highly alcohol-abusive Indian community in British Columbia, Robinson et al[11] screened all children under age 19, and found FAS and FAE to be present in 190 out of every 1,000. This is by far the highest rate recorded in modern literature, but one must keep in mind that it was an isolated, very problem-dominated community.

• Finally, a nationwide birth certificate study of all birth defects done in the U.S. by Chavez et al for the U.S. Centers for Disease Control[4] found FAS to be diagnosed more frequently in American Indian children than among other groups. The rates were: Indians, 29.9 per 1,000; African Americans 6.0 per 1,000; Non-Hispanic whites 0.9 per 1,000; and Hispanics 0.8 per 1,000. Chavez et al,[4] however, expressed concern that FAS may be more frequently diagnosed in minority groups and not recognized or under-diagnosed among Whites. Bray and Anderson have also raised the issue of differential reporting as a possibility in Canada.[3]

• The most widely accepted FAS prevalence rate for the entire U.S. population is 2.2 per 1,000 births[1] with FAE affecting at least another 2.2 per 1,000. Therefore, the most rigorous studies of FAS and FAE among Indians show some communities with similar rates to the overall U.S., while others are higher and some substantially higher.

6. FAS and FAE prevention programs have been operative in a few Indian communities and some are reported to be effective.[5,6,7,8] Those that combine baseline screening for FAS and FAE prevalence with a wide range of primary, secondary, and tertiary prevention programs are believed to be very promising.[5,10] Post-test prevalence studies, however, will need to be done to verify success.

7. Indian communities can effectively carry out programs to prevent the entire range of Alcohol-Related Birth Defects.[8] My experience over the past 12 years has shown that three-way partnerships between tribes, federal agencies, and universities produce a rich mixture of ideas, energies and skill which can be used effectively to prevent ARBD.[5,7,9]

REFERENCES

[1] Abel, E. L. and Sokol, R. J. Incidence of fetal alcohol syndrome and economic impact of FAS-related anomalies. **Drug and Alcohol Depend.** 19:51-70, 1987.

[2] Asante, K. O. and Nelms-Matzke, J. Survey of children with chronic handicaps and fetal alcohol syndrome in the Yukon and Northwest B.C. Ottawa: **Health and Welfare Canada** (unpublished report), 1985.

[3] Bray, D. L. and Anderson, P. D. Appraisal of the epidemiology of fetal alcohol syndrome among Canadian Native peoples. **Can. J. Pub. Hlth.**, 80:42-45, 1989.

[4] Chavez, G. F.; Cordero, J. F.; and Becerra, J. E. Leading major malformations among minority groups in the U.S., 1981-86. **MMWR**, 37(55-3):17-24, 1988.

[5] Masis, K. B. and May, P. A. A Comprehensive local program for the prevention of fetal alcohol syndrome. **Pub. Hlth. Rpts.** 106(5):484-489, 1991.

[6] May, P. A. Alcohol and drug misuse prevention programs for American Indians: Needs and opportunities. **J. Stud. Alcohol**, 47(3):187-195, 1986.

[7] May, P. A. and Hymbaugh, K. J. A pilot project on fetal alcohol syndrome among American Indians. **Alcohol Hlth. Res. World**, 7 (2):3-9, 1983.

[8] May, P. A. and Hymbaugh, K. J. A macro-level fetal alcohol

syndrome prevention program for Native Americans and Alaska Natives: Description and evaluation. **J. Stud. Alcohol**, 50(6):508-518, 1989.

[9] May, P. A.; Hymbaugh, K. J.; Aase, J. M.; and Samet, J. M. Epidemiology of fetal alcohol syndrome among American Indians of the southwest. **Soc. Biol.**, 30:374-387, 1983.

[10] Placier, K. J. Fetal Alcohol Syndrome prevention in American Indian communities of Michigan's upper peninsula. **American Indian and Alaska Native Mental Health Research**, 3(1):16-33, 1989.

[11] Robinson, G. C.; Conry, J. L.; and Conry, R. F. Clinical profile and prevalence of fetal alcohol syndrome in an isolated community in British Columbia. **Can. Med. Assoc**. J. 137:203-207, 1987.

[12] Streissguth, A. P.; Clarren, S. K. and Jones, K. L. Natural history of the fetal alcohol syndrome: A 10-year follow-up of eleven patients. **Lancet**, pp. 85-91, July 13, 1985.

[13] Streissguth, A. P.; Aase, J. M.; Clarren, S. K.; Randels, S. P.; LaDue, R.; and Smith, D. F. Fetal alcohol syndrome in adolescents and adults. **JAMA** 265(15):1961-1967, 1991.

[14] West, J. R. and Goodlett, C. R. Teratogenic effects of alcohol on brain development. **Annals of Medicine**, 22:319-25, 1990.

RECOGNIZING AUTHOR'S POINT OF VIEW

This activity may be used as an individualized study guide for students in libraries and resource centers or as a discussion catalyst in small group and classroom discussions.

The capacity to recognize an author's point of view is an essential reading skill. Many readers do not make clear distinctions between descriptive articles that relate factual information and articles that express a point of view. Think about the readings in Chapter Two. Are these readings essentially descriptive articles that relate factual information or articles that attempt to persuade through editorial commentary and analysis?

Guidelines

1. The following are possible descriptions of sources that appeared in Chapter Two. Choose one of the following source descriptions that best defines each reading in Chapter Two.

Source Descriptions

a. Essentially an article that relates factual information

b. Essentially an article that expresses editorial points of view

c. Both of the above

d. Neither of the above

Sources in Chapter Two

_____ **Source Seven**
"Defining Fetal Alcohol Syndrome and Fetal Alcohol Effect" by Gail Stewart Hand.

_____**Source Eight**
"FAS: A National Crisis" by Robin A. LaDue and Barbara A. VonFeldt.

_____**Source Nine**
"Misdirected Crusade" by Stanton Peele.

_____**Source Ten**
"Disaster on the Reservation" by Tom Daschle and Ben Nighthorse Campbell.

_____**Source Eleven**
"The Situation Is Improving" by Cecelia Firethunder.

_____**Source Twelve**
"FAS Among North American Indians: Overview of Scientific Literature" by Philip A. May.

2. Summarize the author's point of view in one to three sentences for each of the readings in Chapter Two.

3. After careful consideration, pick out one reading that you think is the most reliable source. Be prepared to explain the reasons for your choice in a general class discussion.

CHAPTER 3

FETAL NEGLECT AND SOCIAL RESPONSE

13

FETAL NEGLECT AND
SOCIAL RESPONSE

DRUG-EXPOSED INFANTS:
A GENERATION AT RISK

RosAnn Tetz

RosAnn Tetz is a freelance writer and editor from Silver Spring, Maryland, who specializes in articles on health and religion.

Points to Consider:

1. Describe the effects of cocaine on the unborn child.

2. What is the connection between birthweight and head circumference and learning problems?

3. How might cocaine contribute to a rise in child abuse and neglect?

4. What are the two options in dealing with the issue of cocaine-exposed babies?

5. Why are current drug treatment programs unsuccessful in preventing drug-exposed babies?

RosAnn Tetz, "Crack Babies: An Explosive Crisis," **ICPA Dispatch International,** 1991. Reprinted by permission.

***No one so far knows how to undo the damage
caused by a pregnant crack user.***

The existence of drug-exposed babies is not new. What is new
is the number. Hospitals are reporting rates three to four times
higher than in 1985. Of the thousands of babies exposed to drugs
in the womb, most were subjected to cocaine. Hospitals are frequently seeing repeats now — mothers who year after year come
in to deliver babies and who are still using cocaine.

Cheap, widely available, and fiercely addictive, this smokable
cocaine derivative has become increasingly popular with women.
The use of cocaine by women increased 60 percent from 1982 to
1985. "For women in particular, some of the properties of cocaine
have made it a big drug of choice. There are no needles; you
don't slur your words; it's slimming — you take coke, and you
don't want to eat."

Women often use drugs to escape situations they feel powerless
to change. According to Gloria Weissman of the National Institute
on Drug Abuse (NIDA), women who abuse drugs have more problems than drug-abusing men. They have lower levels of self-
esteem and higher levels of depression and anxiety. They have
more social and economic problems. Even after treatment, 72
percent are unemployed.

PREGNANT WOMEN

Whatever the reason for the rapid growth of crack use among
women, its effects can be especially devastating for pregnant
women and their unborn children. "The word on the street is that if
you smoke lots of crack, you'll have a miscarriage," said Trish
Magyari, director of a March of Dimes prenatal substance-abuse
education program in Washington, D.C. "Sometimes that works
and sometimes it doesn't, but the risk to the baby is severe retardation."

In addition women who use crack tend to use other drugs as
well. They often take alcohol, sedatives, and other downers to
ease the crash that follows a crack high. And few such heavy
drug users get adequate prenatal care. When a woman on crack
gets pregnant, the last thing she is thinking about is the care of the
developing fetus, let alone care of herself. Often the first time a
pregnant crack addict visits a doctor is when she goes into labor
and is ready to deliver — and sometimes not even then.

Many women believe the placenta protects the fetus from the harmful effects of the drugs they take. Researchers say the opposite is true with cocaine: the placenta acts as a sponge, absorbing the drug. Once cocaine enters the fetus's blood and tissues, it circulates much longer than it does in adults. The baby's liver is not yet developed enough to detoxify quickly. And using cocaine even once can have tragic consequences.

If used during the early months of pregnancy, cocaine can cause miscarriage. Used later in pregnancy, it can induce contractions which may cause the baby to be born much too early. Cocaine use can also lead to a condition called *abruptio placentae*, in which the placenta pulls away from the wall of the uterus before labor begins. This can lead to extensive bleeding and can be fatal for both the mother and her baby.

BIRTH DEFECTS

Babies exposed to cocaine in the womb are at an increased risk for birth defects. This damage all seems to result from a reduction in the flow of blood to some particular organ or tissue. The most common defects are malformations involving the urinary tract and the genitals. These infants are also more at risk for kidney problems, heart defects, and seizures. They have a much greater than normal chance of dying of sudden death syndrome (SIDS).

Many of these babies may carry the virus for acquired immune deficiency syndrome (AIDS) and other infectious diseases. They often must be treated for syphilis, which was rare five years ago. Many women addicts resort to prostitution, staying day and night in crack houses, exchanging sex for as little as a single smoke. The rampant trade in sex for crack has apparently contributed to the sudden resurgence of syphilis and has health officials worried about the spread of AIDS among crack users.

Babies exposed to cocaine before they are born may start life with serious health problems. Many are born too soon or too small, sometimes weighing as little as two pounds. Experts estimate that in big city hospitals 50 to 70 percent of premature infants have cocaine in their urine when they are born. These babies are probably born prematurely because cocaine can cause the uterus to contract.

Cocaine produces extreme fluctuations in both the mother's and baby's heart rate and blood pressure. A sudden rise in blood

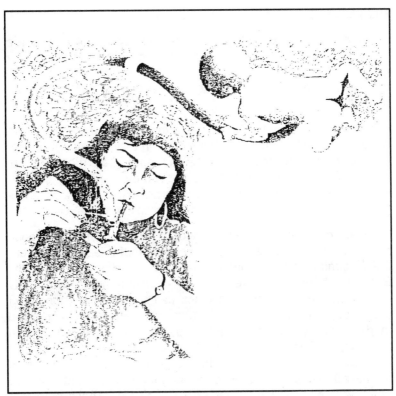

Illustration by Craig MacIntosh. Reprinted by permission of the **Star Tribune,** Minneapolis.

pressure can rupture the tiny, delicate blood vessels in the baby's brain, causing a stroke and irreversible brain damage. If the blood vessels leading to the placenta are constricted even intermittently, the fetal brain is deprived of oxygen, leading to more subtle neurological damage.

Cocaine slows the flow of nutrients and oxygen to the developing body and brain. The diminished blood supply can result in newborns with smaller than normal head size, which may indicate a smaller brain and developmental disabilities. The average reduction of head circumference in babies exposed to cocaine throughout pregnancy is about three-quarters of an inch. The reduction in birth weight is about 21 ounces. These differences are significant. They have been clearly linked to later learning problems and an increased risk of infant mortality...

POVERTY

You can imagine what happens when a baby this difficult to care for is placed with a mother who cares for nothing but her drive for cocaine. Many sociologists and pediatricians are convinced that cocaine is contributing to a recent sharp rise in child abuse and neglect.

In many poor neighborhoods more than half of the families are headed by single women. If the mother in a single-parent household becomes addicted to cocaine, the result is often a no-parent household. According to one addict, "The mothers in my generation are using crack. The daughters are using crack. There's going to be no one left to take care of the children."

The children's physical and developmental problems are intensified by a chaotic home life. It is possible that in a good environment cocaine-exposed babies could catch up developmentally. But these babies are rarely in a good environment. In a study comparing preemies born to crack users with other (noncrack) preemies, even at the age of 18 months, after receiving good medical care and educational therapy, the crack children were in bad shape. They did not know how to play. They tended to hit their toys around the room without apparent motive. Their faces appeared joyless and their body language lacked enthusiasm. They were disorganized in everything they did. These problems were probably a result of the neurological damage caused by cocaine...

SOCIAL PROGRAMS & PROBLEMS

There are only a handful of experimental programs designed expressly to deal with the little understood problems of prenatally drug-exposed children. No training program has yet proven to be completely effective for children with these drug-related afflictions. No one so far knows how to undo the damage caused by a pregnant crack user.

The Los Angeles Unified School District is one of the first school systems in the country to search for a way to deal with this new kind of student. The classrooms are staffed by three adults — a doctor, a psychiatric social worker, and a psychologist — assigned to the program part time. . .

Cocaine is not only destroying individual lives; it is overburdening obstetric and pediatric wards and adding to the ever-mounting cost of health care. In some states determination that a newborn has drugs in its system mandates an investigation. At hospitals cases are piling up by the dozen as case workers arrange home inspections and decide which babies must go to foster homes or grandparents and which stay with the mother. More and more infants are simply abandoned by their addicted mothers at the hospital. These "boarder babies" are medically ready to be discharged from the hospital but have no place to go.

Child welfare officials in several major cities, forced to cope with increasing numbers of neglected children from drug-involved families, are sending a growing number of them to facilities that are reminiscent of orphanages of old: long-term residences housing many children. The devastating impact of the drug problem on families and the failure of foster care to provide an adequate solution have created a demand for far more facilities to care for far younger children for much longer periods of time.

A group nursery of this type costs up to $2,500 a month per baby. The Los Angeles pilot education project costs taxpayers $15,000 a year per pupil. The national price tag for looking after the babies born to mothers who abuse an illegal drug is $2.5 billion a year. And the saddest aspect of the suffering and misery of these children's lives is that it is completely preventable.

TREATMENT

As the crack problem worsens, there are only two options: get mothers into treatment programs in time to protect their babies, or be prepared to deal with an epidemic of troubled children. Expectant mothers must be convinced to avoid drugs. But crack addicts are extremely difficult to work with. They don't want to participate. Drop-out rates are higher than 50 percent.

According to Shirley Coletti, president of a program called Operation Parental Awareness and Responsibility, "We've worked with women with alcohol and heroin problems. Often the maternal instinct of those women has overpowered the drug. They've stayed clean through pregnancy. But with crack they're unable to do that. It's the nature of the drug; it's so potent and powerfully addictive. Crack always wins."

This grim outlook may have some explanation in the fact that pregnant women get short shrift when it comes to drug treatment. Although at least half of crack addicts are now believed to be female, drug treatment is still predominantly a male world. Most of the treatment programs are still based on what the researchers call a male model. The usual approach involves constant confrontation, very possibly the most counter-productive process with women who have exceedingly low self-esteem.

A survey of 78 New York treatment programs found that 54 percent excluded pregnant women and 87 percent excluded crack addicts. If a pregnant woman goes to a treatment facility, chances are it will not accept her. . .

There are no easy answers. But we cannot ignore the problem. The crack babies are here. We must deal with the disabilities and problems that they must live with throughout their lives. The addicted mothers are here — so consumed by their need for crack that they have lost many of their human qualities. We must give them every opportunity to receive treatment to break the bonds of addiction. A new generation of young women is here. We must convince them to stay away from drugs. But ultimately, the only solution is to eliminate the conditions that lead young women to use cocaine.

14

FETAL NEGLECT AND
SOCIAL RESPONSE

LITTLE LASTING HARM
FOR CRACK CHILDREN

Debra Viadero

Debra Viadero wrote the following article for Education Week.

Points to Consider:

1. Summarize Dr. Chasnoff's findings concerning cocaine-exposed children.

2. Explain the significance: "Cocaine use rarely occurs in a vacuum."

3. What other factors might be responsible for babies' impairment?

4. To what does Dr. Chasnoff attribute the increasing number of school-age children with problems?

Debra Viadero, "New Research Finds Little Lasting Harm for 'Crack' Children," **Education Week,** January 29, 1992. Reprinted by permission.

Children whose mothers used cocaine during pregnancy can be better off than was previously thought.

The widely held belief that children born to cocaine-using mothers are forming a permanently damaged "biological underclass" may be largely a myth, according to a growing number of researchers in the field.

New studies published in medical and psychiatric journals, and some that are now in press, suggest that, for the most part, young children who were exposed to cocaine in the womb appear to have a few impairments distinct from those common among children born of poverty.

These researchers say that while many cocaine-exposed children may require a little extra attention once they reach school, the majority of this population, once labeled a "lost generation", will not require full-fledged special-education services.

"What we are finding is that, over all, these children are not retarded," said Ira Chasnoff, a Northwestern University medical researcher who has followed a group of 300 such children since 1986. "Over all, they're within the normal developmental range, and a great majority — at least 70 percent — of the kids are mainstreamed and doing well in general public education."

Dr. Chasnoff, who did some of the earlier work identifying problems among cocaine-exposed children, will publish his newest findings in the *Journal of Pediatrics.*

He said in an interview that he has found that, at ages three, four, and five, more than 90 percent of the cocaine-exposed children enrolled in a special early-intervention program he directs continue to test "within the normal range" on standard intelligence and cognitive tests.

About 30 to 40 percent of the children in the study continue to display delays in language development or problems in concentrating and focusing attention, according to Dr. Chasnoff, who is also president of the National Association for Perinatal Addiction Research and Education.

"THE INCONSOLABLES"

Earlier studies by Dr. Chasnoff and other researchers, in con-

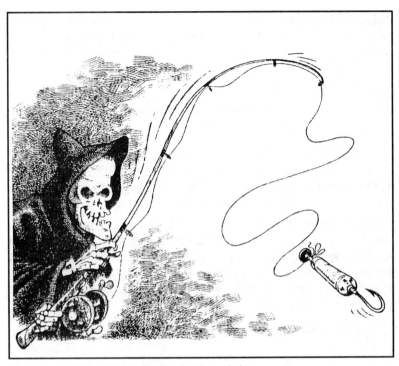

Illustration by Richard Wright. Reprinted with permission.

trast, pointed to much greater problems for these children. (See *Education Week*, Oct. 25, 1989.)

They suggested that cocaine-exposed babies stood a greater risk of being born prematurely or with anatomical malformations. At birth, such children were found to be smaller and weigh less than other infants and had small head circumference — a characteristic, experts say, that is often a marker for developmental disabilities. The studies suggested cocaine-exposed children also were prone to neurological damage, seizures, and sudden infant death syndrome.

In the hospital nursery, the earlier research found, these children, known as "the inconsolables", were often highly irritable, shrinking from the caresses that might calm other infants. At age two, one follow-up study indicated, the children still had problems interacting with others, concentrating, and coping with an unstructured environment. . .

MULTIPLE CAUSES

Even without special help, however, children whose mothers used cocaine during pregnancy may be better off than was previously thought. The problem with the earlier studies is that they failed to take into account other factors that might have contributed to these children's medical problems.

For instance, they note, cocaine use rarely occurs in a vacuum. Mothers who use cocaine are also likely to have used alcohol, tobacco, marijuana, and other harmful drugs during pregnancy. And few studies controlled for that possibility.

"Many people noticed a lot of problems in children and said, 'Aha, cocaine,'" said Claire D. Coles, the director of clinical and developmental research at the human-genetics laboratory at Emory University. "They didn't control for babies being born preterm, sexually transmitted diseases, drugs, the effects of poverty, poor medical care, lifestyle."

"It is a combination of factors that is causing the problems," she said.

Newer studies by Ms. Coles and other researchers have begun to plug in some of the gaps in previous research. As a result, they are finding that, in infants at least, cocaine by itself has had a much smaller effect than some of the previous studies indicated.

A soon-to-be-published study by Ms. Coles of 178 cocaine-exposed infants linked the drug only to lower birthweight and smaller head circumferences in the newborns studied.

"In the absence of other complicating factors, like preterm birth, such infants do not appear to be otherwise impaired physically or behaviorally in the neonatal period," the study concludes.

"Most of this in the [news]paper is just made up out of whole cloth," Ms. Coles said. "The vast majority of the children are fine, and many others, given an adequate environment, are fine, too."

"DEGREES OF RISK"

A similar study published recently by Nancy Day, a University of Pittsburgh researcher, found "no effect whatsoever" of moderate cocaine use by the mothers of 300 newborns studied. Ms. Day said another study in which she is participating, which includes

600 infants whose mothers used the drug more frequently, also suggests maternal cocaine use has had little effect on infants.

"A woman should avoid exposure to any chemical during pregnancy, but there are degrees of risk," said Donald Hutchings, the editor of the *Journal of Neurotoxicology and Teratology* which is publishing some of the new studies.

In terms of physiological effects and sheer prevalence, for example, alcohol may turn out to be a far more dangerous drug for unborn children, according to the researchers.

NEWS MEDIA, EXPERTS FAULTED

The researchers said the attention surrounding the earlier studies has led to exaggerated perceptions about the outlook for cocaine-exposed children. They say the publicity about the problem, illustrated in newspaper headlines calling the children "crack babies" and labeling them "born to lose" or a "generation of sociopaths", has led to widespread perceptions that these children are doomed to fail in school.

"Teachers are already assuming they are problem children and will treat them differently," said Ms. Day, who is an associate professor of psychiatry and epidemiology at the University of Pittsburgh. "Unless we step back and look at the root causes of their problems, we can't cure them. . ."

Some researchers also accuse the popular media of painting a much grimmer picture of the situation than was indicated even by the earlier studies.

Ms. Coles said the exaggerations were easy to believe, in part because the epidemic of "crack" cocaine use that began in the mid-1990s has affected primarily poor, inner-city blacks. "It's easy for society to say, 'This is going on with people who are not like the rest of us,'" she said.

But Mr. Hutchings of the *Journal of Neurotoxicology and Teratology* lays some of the blame at the feet of the professionals in the field. "A lot of this information has come right from clinicians' mouths," he said. "They invited reporters into the nursery and showed them very sick children who were portrayed as 'crack babies'."

Added Ms. Day of the University of Pittsburgh: "I think the politicians also distorted it, because it's easier to attack cocaine than poverty."

LARGER PROBLEM

Despite the hyperbole surrounding cocaine-exposed youngsters, the researchers caution, one aspect of public perception about the problem has been on target: There are growing numbers of children entering school who have more health and behavioral problems than ever before.

An estimated 375,000 children are born exposed to drugs each year, according to one conservative estimate. But the number of children who may need some extra attention in school because they are hungry or homeless, or are being raised by brothers and sisters who are children themselves, among other risk factors, is much larger and growing.

"Their numbers are increasing, not from the drug problem, but from the general environment in which children are being raised today," Dr. Chasnoff said.

"What schools need to do," Ms. Day added, "is stop talking about crack babies and talk about what they've really got — a bunch of kids living in poverty."

"The good news about that," she said, "is that we know how to deal with that."

15   FETAL NEGLECT AND SOCIAL RESPONSE

WE FAIL TO INVEST IN OUR CHILDREN

Charlie M. Knight

Dr. Charlie M. Knight wrote this article in his capacity as the Superintendent of the Ravenwood City School District in East Palo Alto, California.

Points to Consider:

1. Describe the Ravenwood City School District program for drug-affected children.

2. What do drug-exposed babies need most of all, and why is it so difficult to provide?

3. Why do existing public school programs fail to teach drug-exposed children?

4. What government intervention is recommended by the author?

5. What changes in teacher education are recommended?

Excerpted from testimony by Charlie M. Knight before the House Select Committee on Narcotics Abuse and Control, July 30, 1991.

I cannot help but notice that our state legislature seems increasingly less willing to invest in public education now that the majority of students in California are not Caucasian.

My small school district is already reeling from the first crest of the wave of children who enter with more than the usual disabilities resulting from growing up in poverty. At the same time we see funding eroding even for current programs. I cannot help but notice that our state legislature seems increasingly less willing to invest in public education now that the majority of students in California are not Caucasian.

Last fall, when the House of Representatives passed H. R. 1013 (Special Education reauthorization), it recognized the disproportionate numbers of black children, especially black male children who were being placed into Special Education Programs, and recommended research to find more effective ways to serve this group of traditionally underestimated young people. It also recognized that *in utero* drug exposure could result in increasing numbers of children in need of special services. The House bill contained a section calling for demonstration grants to school districts for intervention programs targeted to these children. The House bill contained no categorical funding for these programs. By the time the bill became P. L. 101-476, that language was gone and the only special funding was for coordinating existing services as part of the program evaluation.

THE THROW-AWAY CHILDREN

On Friday, November 2, 1990, the *Oakland Tribune* reported on a study which found that "one in three young black men in California is either in jail, on probation or on parole." Today's eighteen-year-old black man was in second or third grade in 1980. He was more likely to have been identified as "educationally handicapped" than his Anglo or Hispanic peers. He was more likely to have been retained in a grade than other students. He was more likely to have been suspended. He was, in fact, more likely to have found his public school days to be an experience which alienated and disenfranchised him from the mainstream culture.

It should not have been surprising that in the mid-1980s, when crack cocaine became easily available, it would have met with a large group of thirteen-year-old black boys whose teenage rebel-

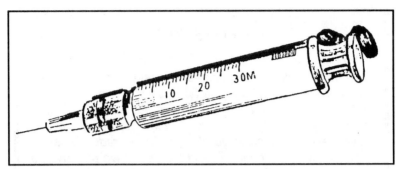

lion was intensified by the low self image they had gained from being told they were failures by their teachers and who had quite reasonably given up on the system for more immediate and tangible rewards. Enter the teenage black girls whose rebellion is made more isolating because their dysfunctional families cannot provide adequate support. As teenagers, these girls face the same pressures toward sex and drugs, and away from school, which are faced by all girls. However, the boys they date are those who have found education to be futile; and the goals of steady job and small house seem vaporous at best when compared to the instant pleasures of sex and drugs.

The mixture has created a new generation of tragedy. The difference is that these least prepared mothers have infants who are extremely frustrating to raise.

If we as a country should have learned anything from the Japanese success, it would have been that our short-sighted view of reality and failure to invest in long-range goals is crippling us today and threatens to destroy us in the future. California's spending on incarceration has increased by more than 500% in stable dollars over the past ten years, while its investment in avoiding incarceration has so eroded that spending on our students places us forty-eighth out of fifty states, and far behind other states with comparable costs of living.

SUCCESS IS POSSIBLE

I have not presented these facts out of bitterness, but out of concern for our future as a nation. We have enough research to be certain that children who are successful in school are unlikely to turn to drugs later, and that the most effective way to control drugs

93

POVERTY

I think drug abuse is added onto the issues of poverty, but I don't think we can address this issue and expect families in poverty to simply give up a drug, whether it is alcohol, cocaine or any other drug without replacing it with something else. I think over the years people in poverty have been expected to go along with the traditional treatment plans and then in the end they still have poverty and no goals, and no future, and things haven't changed.

Maureen E. Montgomery, M.D., Children's Hospital of Buffalo, New York, in testimony before the **Senate Finance Committee,** June 28, 1990

is to eliminate the market for them. It is a "Looking Glass" logic which places enforcement before prevention.

For the past 18 months, the Ravenswood City School District has been running a program for infants and young children born toxic-positive, and their mothers. The program centers around therapeutic day care. Mothers are required to come to the center several times each week for drug and family counseling, parent training, preventive health care, and continuing education. The County's Child Protective Services and Health Departments provide a part-time nurse, a counselor and case management services. Our center serves 44 infants and children and their parents.

From our own early intervention program, funded in part by the Office for Substance Abuse Prevention (OSAP), we have learned that most children who come into this world affected by crack cocaine, can, after even as short a time as 24 months, behave so similarly to non-exposed children as to be indistinguishable. To achieve this level of progress, they need what all children need, a safe, stable, nurturing environment. Their problem is that they enter the world into the most unnurturing environment imaginable, and they would present a challenge to the most experienced and mature of parents. They are agitated and colicky, so they cry often and often fail to provide parents with hugs and smiles, cues which help parents bond with their children. And the parents. . .

The mothers of these difficult children are children themselves, under-educated, immature, without money, and usually without an available supportive family. The fathers are too often the black males who were called "disadvantaged", or "at risk", or "special ed" or any other names that made it acceptable for teachers to give up on them. The fathers are the boys whom we pushed out onto the street, whom we told in a thousand ways that they were too stupid to make it in school. They are the inmates of California's alternative-to-school, its burgeoning prisons. Thus these young girls are left to their own inadequate resources as they raise some of the most difficult children. They have no job skills and little education. It is little wonder that we have found them cutting the ends of the nipples from baby bottles so that they can put broken-up hamburger and lettuce into the bottles. It is little wonder that after being cooped up in a dank apartment with a screaming baby for days at a time, they escape into drugs and loud TV. The result, of course, is the birth and raising of a new generation of American children, malnourished, sickly, and unprepared for an education system which is unable to meet their needs. Instead of leading the United States with their energy and productivity, instead of providing the support our generation will need as we retire, this new generation will become a drain on the country's shrinking resources.

CRACK CHILDREN CAN SUCCEED

The good news is that it is not impossible for us to change this picture. It is not even prohibitively expensive to do so. We have found, and our findings are supported by other programs in the state and around the country, that programs can be developed which will minimize the damage these children suffer and even produce school age youngsters better prepared to succeed in school than many non-drug exposed children. . .

Based on our experiences, I recommend that funds be set aside for grants to school districts from the federal government, perhaps through OSAP. We have found this young agency to be most cooperative and supportive. If funding is routed through the states, a portion must be set aside for programs such as ours, run by local educational agencies.

The total cost of such a program is approximately $12,000 per child per year. By using existing county agency resources, the total cost would be approximately $8,000 per child per year — of which basic child care is about $5,000. At this time, I know of only one other program like ours in California, and as of June it had not begun to enroll children. According to our information, no other

95

school district in the United States has received an OSAP grant — probably because the funding guidelines do not provide for grants which are large enough for the school district to run the program without using its own general funds.

PUBLIC SCHOOL INSTRUCTIONAL PROGRAMS LACK ESSENTIAL ELEMENTS

The greatest weakness of school age programs is that clients have already fallen behind. They have been in an average of three foster care placements; have rotated between mothers and foster care; or have elderly grandparents who have been trying to cope with them. Children's routines have been disrupted, they haven't been able to bond with an adult. They have often suffered from poor nutrition and lack of medical care and have had few pre-education experiences. Identification of children is more difficult. The drug symptoms are now so mixed with the problems of lack of nurturing that the developmental problems require greater skill. This weakness is followed by the lack of a focused family service program which includes health services, counseling, job training and parenting along with the educational interventions for children.

When these vulnerable students arrive in school, they are greeted by teachers who have many children to serve and who often lack both the belief that these children can learn and the skills to effectively instruct them. Further, federal programs for public school children only look at the visible needs of the children. Schools lack the local resources to provide for the children in the context of their families—an essential component to successful intervention. Funding for school-age children must be broad enough to encompass staff development as well as the parenting, counseling and other services we have found to be successful in our Parent-Child Intervention Program (PCIP).

The federal government needs to lead the way in providing holistic programs for school-age children, while concurrently supporting additional research.

TEACHER EDUCATION PROGRAMS IGNORE THE PROBLEM'S EXISTENCE

There is little doubt that new teachers in our state are entering their profession unequipped to teach minority students, let alone drug-affected students. Funding for teacher education programs must require direct experience in urban schools, and must require teacher candidates to participate in both cultural orientations and classwork in dealing with disabilities. These classes in turn must be taught by practitioners who are familiar with the manifestations of drugs and the dysfunctional environments of children.

16

FETAL NEGLECT AND
SOCIAL RESPONSE

MORE SPENDING WON'T
FIX THE PROBLEM

Harmeet K. D. Singh

Harmeet K.D. Singh wrote the following article as an assistant editor of Policy Review. Policy Review *is the flagship journal of the Heritage Foundation, a conservative thinktank in Washington, D.C.*

Points to Consider:

1. How does the behavior and motivation of mothers negate D.C.'s efforts to lower infant mortality?

2. Compare the District of Columbia's infant mortality rate with the national rate. Compare with Japan's rate.

3. What is the goal of WIC, and why is it limited in reducing infant mortality?

4. What is the relationship of illegitimacy to infant mortality?

Harmeet K. D. Singh, "Why American Infants Are Dying," **Policy Review**, Spring, 1990. Reprinted by permision.

A black infant born in the District of Columbia is more likely to die before the age of one than a baby born in North Korea or Bulgaria.

It is a tragedy and a source of embarrassment that the U.S. ranks 20th in the world in preventing infant mortality. Singapore and Hong Kong, as well as Japan and most of Western Europe, all do better. The statistics are particularly bad for minority children: A black infant born in the District of Columbia is more likely to die before the age of one than a baby born in North Korea or Bulgaria. These shameful statistics persist despite the 93 federal programs and $7 billion a year that the country spends to keep children alive.

THE MOTHERS

Most thinking about infant mortality focuses on ways to provide medical insurance for the one-sixth of all women who are both uninsured and ineligible for Medicaid or to deliver health care in their own neighborhoods to women who might be intimidated by hospitals or clinics.

But these proposals fail to address the most important reason for America's high infant mortality: the behavior and motivation of mothers themselves. The situation in the District of Columbia exemplifies the problem. The mayor has bragged that Washington's infant mortality campaign is "the most comprehensive anywhere in the country," and he is probably correct. In D.C., prenatal care is free to any woman whose family income is less than $20,000. Eleven of the city's 16 health clinics provide prenatal care and are required to give a woman an appointment within two weeks (two months is the average in many states). Convenient evening hours make it even easier for women to reach a clinic, and child care is also available. At the clinic, a woman can see an obstetrician, a nurse, a WIC [Special Supplemental Feeding Program for Women, Infants and Children] worker, a social worker, even a dentist, and also be referred for drug treatment.

BETTER BABIES

D.C. has marketed its services well. A highly visible media campaign, called "Better Babies", has posted ads on buses and posters, and broadcast them on television and radio around the

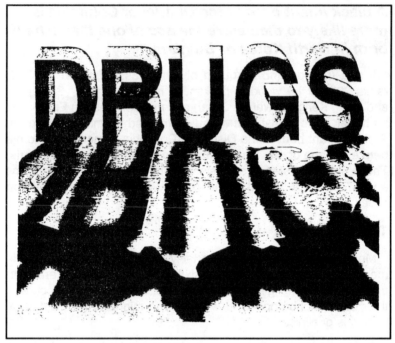

Source: General Accounting Office

city. The MOM van (Maternity Outreach Mobile project) makes the rounds of the city's poorest neighborhoods every day, finding pregnant women, reminding them of their appointments and getting them there if they have no transportation. Nor are private practitioners in short supply: Unlike many other areas of the country, D.C. has plenty of obstetrical care providers, many of whom cater to the Medicaid clientele and are conveniently located throughout the city. Altogether, D.C. spends $105 million on its residents' health.

Despite all of this lavish attention, the District of Columbia has the nation's worst infant mortality rate, 27 per 1,000 in early 1989, or nearly three times the national rate. (In 1988, 10,514 babies were born in D.C.)

OTHER CITIES

Other cities with equally costly infant mortality programs are achieving equally dismal results. Infant mortality in Detroit is almost as bad as in D.C., even though the city employs, at considerable expense, teams of specially trained paraprofessional out-reach workers to comb neighborhoods, find pregnant women and bring them into the public health system. Hartford, Conn., has offered similarly liberal prenatal care for poor women, yet only a third of its teenage mothers sought care in their first trimester.

Why don't women in D.C. and other cities take advantage of the prenatal care offered to them? Clearly, neither lack of availability nor insufficient outreach is the answer. "Most of the women I come into contact with know they can get free care, but a lot of them don't really take prenatal care all that seriously. Some of them say they didn't even know they were pregnant until pretty late in the pregnancy," reports one D.C. public health official.

SUBSTANCE ABUSE

Another explanation for high infant mortality rates lies in the staggeringly high number of babies born to substance-abusing women. Ethel Hawkins, director of social services at D.C. General Hospital, estimates that "well over 60% of the babies born here are born to women who used drugs or alcohol while they were pregnant." Another health care worker placed the toll closer to 70%.

Even when these women are identified and counseled early in the pregnancy, convincing them to stop destroying their children often proves impossible, as the Infant Mortality Research Program of the Department of Agriculture — which identifies pregnant women in D.C. by going door to door in half the city's wards and distributing information in grocery stores and laundromats — has found. According to the program's director, Lilly Munroe-Lord, "It's very difficult to get through to the women who are using crack while pregnant. They simply don't hear you. The ones who are casual users can be convinced to stop during the remainder of the pregnancy, but they usually go right back to it after the baby is born."

BEHAVIOR

Dr. George Graham, professor of human nutrition at Johns Hopkins University, confirms these observations from the field: "I don't know how spending more on prenatal care is going to make any difference to the woman who uses crack. A recent study found that nearly 30% of the babies born in New York hospitals were addicted to crack. Use of drugs, not poor nutrition, is the

> *Infant mortality in Detroit is almost as bad as in D.C., even though the city employs, at considerable expense, teams of specially trained paraprofessional outreach workers to comb neighborhoods, find pregnant women and bring them into the public health system. Hartford, Conn., has offered similarly liberal prenatal care for poor women, yet only a third of its teenage mothers sought care in their first trimester.*

leading cause of low birthweight. You hear a lot about how nutritional deficiencies, lack of funds for WIC, etc., are responsible for low birthweight, but that's simply false. Low birthweight in the U.S. is not caused by poor feeding programs — it's usually caused by the behavior of the mother."

Teen pregnancy and illegitimacy are also important causes of low birthweight and infant mortality. American Enterprise Institute researcher Nicholas Eberstadt recently wrote in a nationally syndicated column, "If viewed as a medical condition, illegitimacy would be one of the leading killers of children in America." Mr. Eberstadt's work suggests that a child born to poor, married parents has a better chance of survival than a child born to a middle-class single mother: Infant mortality rates, according to one 1982 study, can be higher for children of unmarried white college graduates than for children of married white high-school dropouts.

Not so coincidentally, D.C., which trails the nation in infant mortality, also has the nation's highest percentage of births to unmarried mothers. Fifty-eight percent of all babies in the city are born to unmarried women — nearly three times the national average.

CONCLUSION

Responsible maternal behavior may even compensate for comparatively poorer prenatal care. A Japanese woman is four times more likely to die during childbirth than an American woman, because complex medical treatment is more likely to be available here. Yet Japan has the world's lowest rate of infant mortality — about half that of the U.S. In Japan, fewer than 1% of all mothers are either unmarried or teenagers.

America's high rate of infant mortality is more of a social problem than a medical problem. Spending more won't fix it.

17   FETAL NEGLECT AND SOCIAL RESPONSE

BOARDER BABIES: ABANDONED IN THE CRIB

Shirley E. Marcus

Shirley E. Marcus is the deputy director of the Child Welfare League of America (CWLA), a membership organization of more than 670 child serving agencies comprised of both public and private non-profit providers serving children and their families.

Points to Consider:

1. Provide an estimate of the number of boarder babies in the United States.

2. What is the range of cost per day for a boarder baby?

3. Why are welfare workers struggling to find permanent, loving homes for boarder babies?

4. What difficulties might adoptive parents face?

5. How might judicial reform help the plight of boarder babies?

Excerpted from testimony by Shirley E. Marcus before the House Committee on Education and Labor, Subcommittee on Select Education, May 28, 1992.

A shocking 85 percent of the boarder babies in our survey were prenatally exposed to either alcohol, illicit drugs, or both.

While most of my remarks will be devoted to the results of a recent boarder baby survey conducted jointly by the Child Welfare League of America (CWLA) and the National Association of Public Hospitals (NAPH), I want to provide a broader context for the numbers I am about to discuss.

For much of the last ten years, the United States has conducted a self-proclaimed "war on drugs". This conflict has produced many casualties. For example:

In 1987, homicide accounted for 42 percent of all deaths to African American males between the ages of 15 and 24. In fact, homicide is the leading cause of death for both African American males and females 15 to 24 years of age. Obviously, many of these cold-blooded murders are directly related to the drug trade.

The National Association of State Alcohol and Drug Directors (NASAD) estimates that 280,000 pregnant women are actively engaged in alcohol abuse, illegal drug use or both simultaneously. However, only 11 percent of these women actually receive treatment of any kind.

The American Public Welfare Association (APWA) estimates that there are now over 407,000 children on any given day in out-of-home placements, which represents a 50 percent increase just since 1986 — the year crack cocaine hit the streets of our Nation's major metropolitan areas. Many of the new entrants into the foster care system are below the age of five.

1) Numbers:

Viewed in this light, it's clear that abandoned infants and boarder babies are simply among the most tragic casualties in our Nation's struggle to overcome an ongoing substance abuse crisis of enormous proportions. Indeed, the startling results of our survey point to the magnitude of the national problem we face. Using a standard definition of an abandoned infant as "any infant who, though medically cleared for discharge, cannot go home because there is neither a biological home nor alternative placement immediately available," the CWLA/NAPH study discovered that 22 hospitals in 12 cities serve a projected annual total of over 6,000

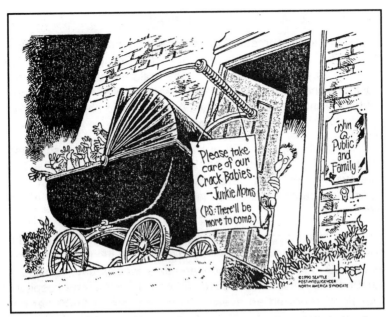

Cartoon by David Horsey. Reprinted with special permission of North American Syndicate.

boarder babies. Since we have information indicating that 119 hospitals nationwide provide care for boarding infants, the actual total is probably several times the projected number contained in our survey.

Not surprisingly, public hospitals located in major metropolitan areas were hardest hit by the boarder baby phenomenon. As an illustration, the New York City Human Services Administration reports that city hospitals serve an average of 357 boarder babies per month or a total exceeding 4,200 per year. At the same time, just four public hospitals in Los Angeles provide care for almost 1,000 infants who are abandoned or are boarding. Similarly, an estimated 300 infants a year are housed in three hospitals in Chicago. Yet perhaps the most surprising results come from municipalities like Cleveland. Even though that city is less than half the size of Chicago, two hospitals there serve over 125 boarder babies per year.

2) Characteristics/Cost:

A closer look at the characteristics of these children gives an inkling of the difficulties confronted by child welfare agencies both in terms of keeping infants with their families or providing an appropriate foster or adoptive placement.

A shocking 85 percent of the boarder babies in our survey were prenatally exposed to either alcohol, illicit drugs, or both. The most common illegal substance the children are exposed to is crack cocaine. Another 8 percent presented with a developmental delay or disability at birth. Only 2 percent of the children identified by the CWLA/NAPH survey were HIV positive.

Although the human cost of HIV infection or prenatal substance exposure is strikingly high, the financial burden on the public hospital system and child welfare agencies is also substantial. The figures we gathered on hospital boarding rates revealed a wide variation.

Flint, Michigan reported the lowest board rate of $200 per day; hospital facilities in Los Angeles indicated that it can cost as much as $1,800 to house an abandoned infant for one day. Obviously, length of stay also affects cost. As an illustration, one hospital in Cleveland reported an average boarding rate of $600 per day. However, since one infant has stayed at that same hospital for five months, the total boarding charge for the child exceeded $90,000. The New York Human Resources Administration estimates that New York City might spend as much as $3.5 million per day to house their boarding infants. We estimated that it might cost as much as $5 million per day to care for the 6,000 infants we identified in the hospital system.

Moreover, these infants strain the resources of hospitals in a variety of ways. During the course of the survey, we discovered one hospital in Miami that converted offices and classrooms into temporary nurseries in order to accommodate the ten to fifteen boarder babies they serve per month.

Please note that once an infant is medically cleared for discharge, Medicaid ceases to pay for the child's care. Under normal circumstances, county government reimburses for only part of the expense, or the hospital's costs go completely uncompensated.

3) Permanency Planning/Developmental Status:

The ultimate placement goal for all children in the child welfare system should be a permanent, loving home, either with one's own family or through adoption. Tragically, this is too often not the case today, because the child welfare system is simply overwhelmed.

HIDDEN PROBLEM

No one knows how many abandoned babies we are dealing with because the federal government does not collect these statistics and in many communities the problem is hidden because of public outrage at babies boarding in hospitals for months and even years.

William L. Pierce, President of the National Council for Adoption in testimony before the **House Committee on Education and Labor**, May 28, 1992

The 50 percent rise in foster care caseloads that I mentioned earlier has occurred at the same time the number of foster homes fell by 34 percent. Further, the AIDS epidemic and the upward spiral in substance abuse have caused these children to enter foster care with physical and emotional needs unimaginable just a decade ago. The complexity of children's cases makes placement in foster care all the more difficult as foster parents must be recruited and trained to care for these children. The severity of the crisis has also contributed to delays in moving children out of foster care, as caseworkers work feverishly to "triage" the most urgent cases and leave others to languish in temporary placements.

Given the present dearth of resources, overburdened child welfare workers are wrestling with the ethics of permanently severing biological parents' rights to regain custody of a child when parents have had no opportunity to remedy their chemical dependency problems. Should a mother's right to rear her child be terminated forever, when she has never received access to drug treatment to remedy the condition that necessitated the child's removal from the home? On the other hand, would failure to terminate rights violate the child's right to a permanent, safe, loving home?

Compounding the dilemma, adoptive homes willing and able to care for children with special needs are in as short supply as foster homes. As many as 31,000 children have had parental rights terminated but remain in temporary care; an additional 40,000 children have plans of adoption but parental ties have not yet been cut. Caseworkers are often reluctant to initiate termination proceedings when that means that a child could remain in temporary care as long as three to five years before being placed in an adoptive home.

Especially in regard to drug-exposed infants, prospective adoptive parents may be anxious about the long-term effects of exposure and the possible need for expensive medical, educational, and psychological care. In addition, without support services to maintain a child in an adoptive home, there is no guarantee that a finalized adoption will be a permanent solution for the child. Nationwide, as many as 13 percent of adoptions disrupt.

Such are the realities of securing permanent homes for boarder babies. Information provided by the hospitals we surveyed provides an illustration of the variety of solutions that are being attempted on behalf of these children. As might be assumed, hospitals who participated in our survey expected to place nearly 75 percent in out-of-home care but a surprising 21 percent of these children were expected to be reunited with their birth parents. Finally, hospitals calculated that only five percent would be freed immediately for adoption. However, the time frame covered by the CWLA/NAPH was only a few months; that figure probably radically understates the number of boarder babies who eventually are adopted.

Moreover, because the condition of drug-exposed infants cannot be predicted, some agencies prefer to place a child in temporary foster care for several months to assess the extent of his injury. While 85 percent of the infants in our survey were drug-exposed, just eight percent of the boarder babies in our survey presented with immediate developmental disabilities at birth ranging from mental retardation to cerebral palsy. In addition, the most recent research indicates that drug and alcohol-exposed infants exhibit a wide array of difficulties ranging from irritability and irregular sleep patterns to tremulousness and hypersensitivity to light and touch. In many ways, the physical symptoms are the most troubling.

Some of the cocaine-exposed infants — who are often in the greatest distress — are extremely jittery and have increased muscle tone which, in turn, leads to delayed motor development and practical difficulties like feeding problems. Nevertheless, a child who is stiff, screams inconsolably, and has projectile vomiting at two months may have recovered almost completely at five months. Conversely, a child without overt symptoms of drug withdrawal at two months may exhibit substantial developmental disabilities at seven months. A child who tests positive for HIV at birth may or may not develop full-blown AIDS.

While such conditions may or may not persist as the child matures, prospective adoptive parents have a right to be fully informed about the extent of their life-long responsibilities if they decide to welcome such a child into their home.

4) Expediting Placement of Abandoned Infants:

Clearly, overcoming barriers to the permanent placement of abandoned infants — and all children in the child welfare system — is in urgent need of leadership, but in the view of the Child Welfare League of America, simply imposing stringent deadlines for termination of parental rights will not accomplish this goal.

In short, boarder babies need a good deal more than well-meaning foster or adoptive parents. Alcohol and drug problems are amenable to prevention and remediation when appropriate services are provided. Child welfare agencies need to expand and enhance services to strengthen and support chemically dependent families to allow them, when in the child's best interests, to retain or regain custody of their children.

When a child must be removed from his or her biological parents, child welfare agencies have a responsibility to engage in an intensive effort to recruit and train foster and adoptive parents to address the specialized needs of these children. Moreover, among an array of family support services is frequent respite care due to the relatively high burn out rate of foster families who care for drug-exposed infants. Finally, a full range of in-home developmental services should be provided including occupational therapy, physical therapy, speech-language therapy and other specialized health care services.

I do not mean to imply that judicial reform can be ignored. That a child will secure a permanent home without delay once his case reaches the court is very unlikely in most states, since the courts are faced with the same shortage in personnel and explosion of cases as state agencies. Steps must be taken to improve decision making by the courts and the legal system through training and supportive services that ensure understanding of child welfare law, alcohol and drug issues, and sensitivity to the needs of children and chemically involved families.

In addition, state governments must review current laws governing the grounds, as well as the time frames for termination of parental rights, to assure that artificial time frames, do not serve as barriers to individualized decision making but that children for whom termination is the clear and best solution are attended to without delay.

5) In Conclusion

Mandatory timelines are no substitute for the resources required by courts and child welfare agencies across the country to speed the transition of abandoned infants from inappropriate hospital settings, while assuring high quality adoptive and foster placements. CWLA hopes for a political bipartisan consensus and the leadership that our children so desperately need to live safe, healthy, secure lives. We strongly urge that as Congress continues the difficult work of allocating scarce federal resources, your most vulnerable constituents, children in the child welfare system, will not be forgotten.

18   FETAL NEGLECT AND SOCIAL RESPONSE

MOST BOARDER BABIES ARE NOT ABANDONED

Cecilia Zalkind

Cecilia Zalkind is the Assistant Director of the Association for Children for New Jersey (ACNJ). ACNJ has advocated for the children of New Jersey for over 140 years. Originally founded as the Newark Orphan Asylum in 1847, ACNJ has become the major independent child advocacy organization in New Jersey. The board, staff and members work on a broad range of issues affecting children, including child abuse, foster care, adoption, child care, education, juvenile justice, homelessness and legal rights for children.

Points to Consider:

1. In what sense have parents not voluntarily left their children in the hospital?

2. Why does the "risk assessment" process delay the discharge of boarder babies?

3. What is the concept of "permanency", and how might the legal process of freeing children for adoption be improved?

4. If the state's obligation is to assist families to stay together, what service should be provided?

Excerpted from testimony by Cecilia Zalkind before the House Committee on Education and Labor, Subcommittee on Select Education, May 28, 1992.

Most "boarder babies" are not abandoned by their parents in the traditional sense of abandonment.

The needs of children in the child welfare system have been a longstanding priority of our advocacy efforts. We believe that our experience can provide the committee some insight in three critical areas:

Defining "abandoned infants" or "boarder babies"

Ensuring timely permanency planning for children in foster care

Achieving appropriate service development

BENEATH THE LABELS OF "ABANDONED INFANTS" AND "BOARDER BABIES"

In 1991, the New Jersey Hospital Association conducted a survey of the hospitals in the state with pediatric or obstetric care units to determine the nature and extent of the boarder baby problem—those newborns or children ready for medical discharge but who remain in hospital care because they have nowhere else to go. The survey found that there were 311 boarder babies and children in New Jersey hospitals during the first quarter of 1991, many of whom remained in hospital care a month or longer.

The Hospital Association survey was extremely helpful in calling attention to the problem and in suggesting some recommendations for change. It did not, however, explore the underlying reasons for the delay in planning for these children nor did it examine exactly who these children were and whether or not they were truly abandoned.

The Association for Children of New Jersey (ACNJ), along with the Department of Public Advocate, became interested in following up on these questions and in early 1992 conducted interviews of hospital personnel in 10 hospitals located in the counties with the greatest number of boarder babies and the longest length of time in hospital care. Our preliminary findings, which we plan to publish in a report, and other information we reviewed, suggest some interesting points:

1) *The children who tend to stay the longest in hospital care are drug-exposed infants.* In the hospitals we contacted, over 90% of the children who remain in the hospital after medical discharge are drug-exposed infants. Length of stay beyond medical

discharge is on average six weeks, although some babies do stay longer, some as long as six months.

These infants are not usually children with medical problems. Although drug-exposed, they are not always drug-addicted. They tend not to have severe medical problems or AIDS involvement. In fact, HIV positive babies or infants with medical problems are usually placed quickly in foster homes, since New Jersey has developed a Special Home Service Provider Program which has been extremely successful in developing foster homes for medically fragile children.

2) *The parents have not voluntarily left their children in the hospital.* Our discussions with hospital personnel revealed that the most common reason why babies remain in the hospital after medical discharge is because the hospital has kept the baby pending a protective services investigation by the state child welfare agency. In the hospitals we contacted, identification of drug use by the mother results in an automatic referral to the Division of Youth and Family Services for assessment of risk to the child.

The hospital is able to keep the child by exercising its right under the child protection laws to "hold" the child pending an investigation. This is not parental abandonment — the hospital, in fact, has prevented the parent from leaving the hospital with the baby. In some cases, the parent remains involved and continues to visit the baby in the hospital.

3) *Conducting the risk assessment contributes to the delay in planning.* The assessment of risk to the child is a critical element in planning for the child and appears to contribute significantly to the delay in discharging children from the hospital. We found that although reporting by the hospital and initial response by the child protection agency is conducted in a timely fashion, the actual assessment and development of a case plan takes a great deal of time.

Assessing risk to the child seems particularly difficult for the protective services agency when the parent is drug-involved. Our analysis of this issue has raised some critical questions that need to be considered when deciding whether or not a child can safely be discharged to the care of his or her parent:

• Are there clear standards for how the risk assessment is conducted and what factors must be considered?

• Are child protection workers adequately trained in the special issues of drug-involved families?

• Are relatives identified and assessed as to their ability to provide support to the family or care for the child?

4) *The delay in discharging the baby from the hospital is directly related to the availability of appropriate services.* An important part of the dilemma for child protection workers is the lack of services for drug-involved families. Even if a worker decides that a child can be safely returned home if services are provided, that plan cannot be implemented unless those services are available and accessible. Services for drug-involved women are particularly sparse in our state. For many women, the only way to obtain treatment is through in-patient services, forcing their children to be placed in foster care. If foster care is the plan, the lack of available foster homes can result in a child staying in the hospital for a prolonged period of time until a home is found. New Jersey has had a particularly difficult time recruiting sufficient foster home resources for babies.

In summary, our preliminary findings reveal that most "boarder babies" are not abandoned by their parents in the traditional sense of abandonment. In fact, they tend to spend prolonged stays in the hospital while the social service system attempts to decide what is in their best interests, hampered by a critical lack of appropriate services, services which could enhance and expedite decision-making and permanency for them.

ENSURING TIMELY PERMANENCY PLANNING FOR CHILDREN IN FOSTER CARE

The delay experienced by the child in being discharged from the hospital to the care of a family is only one part of the problem. Once the child enters foster care, delays often continue and permanence for the child is prolonged or not achieved. Our research and advocacy efforts for children in foster care demonstrate that children continue to stay in foster care too long before alternative plans, such as adoption, are considered for them.

ACNJ is a firm believer in the concept of permanency — that every child has the right to a permanent home. We have devoted significant time and energy to identifying and removing barriers to timely decision-making for adoption-potential children. Our 1984 ABA Project on Special Needs Adoption, undertaken in cooperation with the Division of Youth and Family Services, was highly successful in improving the legal process of freeing children for adoption.

What we learned in our project is that too often delays are caused by three general problems: lack of staff and service resources, poor coordination among the courts, attorneys and the child welfare agency and the low priority of children in the court system. We believe that enhancing and improving timely decision-making for children needing adoption could benefit from:

Sufficient staff resources at every level — social service staff, attorneys, judges and court personnel — to handle these cases quickly and appropriately. training for judges in child development and children's needs so that they understand the critical importance of timely, permanent decision-making.

Sufficient services to assist families stay together so that if a child enters placement and cannot return home, there is documentation to support an early determination that termination of parental rights is appropriate.

We would strongly support efforts to ensure that children for whom adoption is the goal are freed for adoption in an expeditious manner. We are concerned, however, about any proposal that emphasizes adoption without sufficient support to birth families first. We believe strongly that the state's obligation is, and must continue to be, to assist families to stay together. Only when those efforts fail should adoption be considered for the child.

This policy has been expressed and recently re-emphasized in our state law. Amendments to New Jersey's termination of parental rights law, adopted in September 1991, require the state agency to make diligent efforts to assist families to stay together before pursuing adoption for the child. Such diligent efforts require the identification of services to keep the family together.

SERVICE AVAILABILITY IS CRITICAL

It is impossible to over-emphasize the critical importance of appropriate, accessible services for children and families at every step of this process. The availability of services impacts directly on the ability of children to stay with their families, to return home promptly should foster care become necessary and to achieve an alternative permanent plan, like adoption, should return home become impossible. How quickly this decision-making process can occur so that children do not linger indefinitely in foster care depends in great part on service availability and delivery.

This is especially critical when parental drug use is involved. Services for drug-involved families in New Jersey are in short supply and, even when available, are not accessible to provide effective assistance for families. There are too few out-patient treatment programs and almost no in-patient programs that accept a parent and child together. Those programs that do exist do not often deal with parenting issues. Further, unless treatment is provided for pregnant women, we will always be dealing with the problem as a crisis.

The Abandoned Infants Assistance Act has enabled states to develop necessary services. Its level of funding, however, is not sufficient to meet the extraordinary needs of these children and families. We are strongly supportive of any efforts to expand funding under this Act.

116

INTERPRETING
EDITORIAL CARTOONS

This activity may be used as an individualized study guide for students in libraries and resource centers or as a discussion catalyst in small group and classroom discussions.

Although cartoons are usually humorous, the main intent of most political cartoonists is not to entertain. Cartoons express serious social comment about important issues. Using graphic and visual arts, the cartoonist expresses opinions and attitudes. By employing an entertaining and often light-hearted visual format, cartoonists may have as much or more impact on national and world issues as editorial and syndicated columnists.

Points to Consider:

1. Examine the cartoon by David Horsey, on page 105.

2. How would you describe the message of the cartoon? Try to describe the message in one to three sentences.

3. Do you agree with the message expressed in the cartoon? Why or why not?

4. Does the cartoon support the author's point of view in any of the readings in this publication? If the answer is yes, be specific about which reading or readings and why.

5. Are any of the readings in Chapter Three in basic agreement with the cartoon?

CHAPTER 4

CRIME, PREGNANCY AND DRUGS

19   CRIME, PREGNANCY AND DRUGS

CRIMINAL ACTION AND PERINATAL DRUG ABUSE: AN OVERVIEW

Judith Larson

Judith Larson is the Specialist Consultant to the Center on Children and the Law, a program of the American Bar Association Young Lawyers Division. As a private attorney, Larson represents children and their families in neglect and abuse cases in the District of Columbia. For the ABA Center on Children and the Law, Larson trains judges and social workers to identify and respond to parental substance abuse issues in child neglect and abuse cases.

Points to Consider:

1. What has parental substance abuse brought to the state courts?

2. Contrast Minnesota's system for controlling pregnant women's drug ingestion with that of Washington and Oregon.

3. Discuss benefits and limitations of drug-testing mothers and newborns.

4. What is the "reasonable efforts" provision of Public Law 96-272, and how is it increasingly being interpreted?

Excerpted from testimony by Judith Larson before the House Committee on Ways and Means, Subcommittee on Human Resources, April 30, 1991.

Perhaps no subject is so charged with emotion as the decision to remove children from their homes.

State child neglect and abuse laws developed over the past two decades tend to contain broad definitions of neglect and abuse that describe how the child welfare agency is to protect the child from immediate harm and develop a permanent, safe home — preferably with the natural family — without undue delay. These state laws tend to be simple and flexible.

From time to time there are waves of anxiety about social issues that bring those laws under state legislative scrutiny. Parental substance abuse is the most recent of these social crises. It has brought to the courts not only unprecedented numbers of neglect and abuse cases but a younger population of victims — and some analysts fear a more intractable family dysfunction than we have seen in the past. Again, we are asking whether the broad definitions of neglect and abuse in the older laws are flexible enough to meet the new crisis, or whether child welfare agencies and courts must be given more precise directions to enable swift identification and protection of children at risk from parental substance abuse.

1. Controlling the mother's behavior during pregnancy.

In its civil neglect and abuse laws, the State of Minnesota has attempted to develop a system for controlling the pregnant woman's ingestion of illegal substances. The system involves reporting her behavior to the local welfare agency, assessing her condition, offering her services, and allowing the local welfare agency to seek civil commitment for drug treatment if the woman refuses proffered services. For the most part, that law is carefully crafted to rest on a professional medical assessment of obstetrical impairment.

Other states have reacted very cautiously to the approach of controlling the mother's behavior through civil laws. Not only is the subject a minefield of constitutional issues, which have not yet been fully explored by the courts, but a number of states have decided that the same goal can be accomplished by fully funding their drug-treatment programs, and giving priority to pregnant women. The experience of states like Washington and Oregon is that pregnant women will voluntarily enter well designed drug-treatment programs if they are available. That legislative experience has been borne out by numerous drug treatment clinics for pregnant women around the country in which admission is volun-

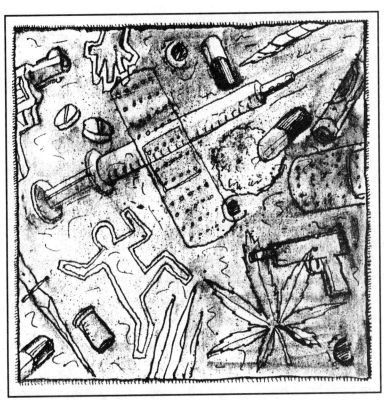

Bulletin of Municipal Foreign Policy

tary and the clinics are always full.

2. Drug-testing a parent or a newborn as a basis for reporting or prosecution.

The broad, inclusive language of state neglect and abuse laws does not, of course, require or recommend drug testing as a way to develop evidence of a substance abuse problem in the dysfunctional family. A number of state legislatures felt the need to provide guidance to its child protection agencies, prosecutors and judiciary on this subject. No doubt it seemed appealing to have a chance to confirm suspicions of a drug problem with what appears to be scientific evidence: actual traces of specific drugs in the body fluids of either a parent or an infant. One overwhelming question has developed, however, in states where statutes were amended specifically to address drug testing:

Does the presence of illegal drugs in body fluids prove, or even

121

indicate, neglect or abuse of a child?

The answer to this question will suggest how the drug tests are to be used. If a positive drug test may prove neglect or abuse, it could be placed in the section of the law which addresses how a case shall be prosecuted. If a positive drug test merely indicates a possibility of neglect or abuse, the test would better fit into the part of the law that describes what kind of behavior must be reported to the child welfare agency.

No state requires drug testing for all newborn infants. In most states, therefore, drug testing of pregnant women and newborn infants is a matter governed by hospital protocols or policies. Many of these rely on social profiles of the women (and some of these profiles correlate with poverty factors like homelessness, uncleanliness and lack of economic support) as well as on medical information about the mother and child, such as weight, nourishment, head circumference, withdrawal symptoms, and so forth.

3. Removing children from their homes and terminating parental rights.

Perhaps no subject is so charged with emotion as the decision to remove children from their homes, whether it occurs early in a case as a protective measure, or later, when the decision to terminate parental rights is being made. Indeed, a pattern of precipitous removal of children was one of the motivations for Congress to enact the "reasonable efforts" provision of Public Law 96-272. The current substance abuse crisis with its high proportion of abandoned babies and low availability of appropriate drug treatment has child welfare administrators and lawmakers wondering whether fast-track, out-of-home placements should not become the norm again. A few states have amended their neglect and abuse and termination of parental rights laws to make early removals easier.

4. Conclusion

At the center, we observe three areas of the law that are particularly vulnerable to change through the insertion of drug-specific language in State laws. Those areas are: First, controlling the behavior of the pregnant woman; second, requiring or permitting the use of positive drug tests, either as a basis for reporting or for prosecuting a neglect case; and third, earlier removal of children from homes and easier termination of parental rights procedures.

Briefly, we find diminishing interest in the States for using the civil neglect and abuse laws to control behavior of the pregnant woman, and this is mirrored on the criminal side by what we view as unsuccessful efforts to do so through the criminal laws.

Instead, we find States looking seriously at putting increased funds into programs for pregnant women and early intervention programs, to attract voluntary compliance. And from what we have seen of those demonstration programs or those private programs in States across the Nation, we have high hopes for success of these efforts, and we applaud them. We note that a number of bills have been or are about to be introduced in this Congress that would increase funding for such programs.

In the second area, the use of positive drug tests, first of all, we would note that Public Law 96-272 places no barrier to the use of a positive drug test as evidence in a neglect case. Furthermore, we would note that those few States, maybe a half dozen, that have amended their laws to permit or require the use of positive drug tests, perhaps equating them to neglect by saying that a parent with a positive drug test is presumptively neglectful, have run into two difficulties.

The first is that it is very difficult to draft a provision that accurately reflects the scientific basis for a positive drug test. There have been linguistic problems in every State. The second is that we are now much more sophisticated than we were, for example, in 1985, and we know that there are limits to what a positive drug test can show us and we know how many children will be missed by using positive drug tests, since the time window is so short. In other words, with cocaine, you would have to have taken drugs 72 hours before the test, in order for it to actually show up, so that those children that you saw in the nursery in Washington, D.C.

might never show positive on a drug test, but still would have been damaged by ingestion of drugs early in the pregnancy.

So, we would see no compelling reason to develop a Federal law that would permit or require the use of positive drug tests, since there are scientific problems with their use, and in any case they are already permitted under Public Law 96-272.

As to the third area, the easier termination of parental rights and earlier removal of children in danger, we would also observe that Public Law 96-272 puts no barrier in front of the social worker or law enforcement officer to removing a child who is immediately in danger. In other words, under the Federal law and under the State laws that reflect those Federal provisions, there is no requirement that if a child is obviously in danger, you must nevertheless leave that child in the home in order to bring in services that would help keep the family together.

So, why is it that children are still dying and are still being injured in homes after reports have been made to the child welfare agency? It is our observation that there are inadequate training and inadequate resources; inadequate training not just of the social worker and the other professionals that immediately come in contact with the child, but also of the judiciary and the lawyers that are involved. They cannot always recognize a substance abuse problem, and thus cannot bring the right resources to bear on it.

The State of Rhode Island had four fatalities last year. The Child Advocate investigated the causes of those fatalities, and in no case was it found that there was a problem with the law. In every case, it was found that there was a problem with inadequate training or inadequate resources.

As far as revising a Federal law to radically change the time within which one must make a decision about a boarder baby, for example, we have grave concerns about moving too quickly in that area. For one thing, Public Law 96-272 again places no barrier to making an early decision about that. There is the 18-month deadline as an outside parameter, but no required waiting period that would prevent swift decisions.

The problem we see is that States are inadequately or differently funded, so that State A may have a lot of resources to bring to bear on making a good early decision about an abandoned baby,

124

but State B may have no resources and end up just being a policing agency that identifies substance-using parents and removes the children. So, what we at the Center on Children and the Law would prefer to see, if Congress is moved in this direction, would be demonstration projects, so then we can scrutinize them and see if there are any problems, before we make any particular changes.

CRIME, PREGNANCY AND DRUGS

WE MUST CRIMINALIZE
FETAL NEGLECT

Paul A. Logli

Paul A. Logli wrote the following article in his capacity as the prosecuting attorney for Winnebago County in Rockford, Illinois. Logli believes that drug-abusing pregnant mothers should be prosecuted.

Points to Consider:

1. Describe the task the writer sets before the State of Illinois Legislature.

2. Explain the analogy between driver education and drug education.

3. What does the writer view as the components of a successful program to protect newborns?

Paul A. Logli in a response to the editor's request for his position on the issue of criminal prosecution of sustance abusing pregnant women, December 1989.

The state must set out a definition of behavior which is so wanton in its disregard for human life and safety that persons engaging in it must be held responsible in the criminal courts.

Recently this office sought to bring charges against a 24-year-old mother as a result of the death of her two-day-old child. According to local medical authorities that death was directly related to the mother's use of cocaine during her pregnancy.

As events turned out, that prosecution was never advanced beyond the Winnebago County Grand Jury due to its decision not to indict the mother who had been previously charged on a police complaint. Thus this case was concluded without a chance to argue important issues before a judge or jury.

SOCIAL CONTROVERSY

In spite of this local setback, it is clear that the case has generated controversy and thought throughout the country. I have personally participated in discussions with numerous concerned individuals in New York, San Diego, Nashville, West Palm Beach, Chicago and Phoenix. It is apparent that the problem of children born either exposed or addicted to alcohol or drugs has become a difficult issue in practically every city and state. In most cases a child exposed or addicted will survive. That triumph, however, is tempered by continuing developmental problems, both physical and mental, that the child will face throughout his lifetime.

ADOPTIVE MOTHER

I received a disturbing and heartbreaking letter from an adoptive mother in the Chicago suburbs. Her adopted child is now four years old and suffers from a multitude of physical problems ranging from cerebral palsy to bone deformities caused by the biological mother's alcohol and drug abuse during the pregnancy.

According to the letter writer, the biological mother was aware of the damage she was doing to her child while still in the womb and in spite of treatment at one of Chicago's prenatal centers for drug abusing pregnant women, the child was still damaged by the use of cocaine and other drugs throughout all stages of the pregnancy. The letter writer states, "my heart breaks for my little girl, who though physically disabled, is intellectually intact as she watches her siblings run and play. She, even at this young age, wonders

127

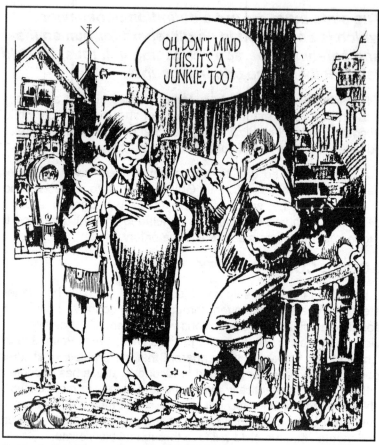

Cartoon by David Seavey. Copyright 1990, **USA Today**. Reprinted with permission.

why she cannot! The truth is, she is a victim of a society that makes laws of convenience."

UNACCEPTABLE BEHAVIOR

Although it isn't convenient or simple, I have called upon the Legislature of the State of Illinois to set about the difficult task of first establishing that the protection of the health of our newborn has to be a priority in the medical, social and legal structures within our state. Secondly, having established this priority, they must work with experts in these areas to set out the boundaries of unacceptable behavior by pregnant women which may constitute a substantial threat to children who survive birth, but who are then captive to serious medical and educational disabilities.

HARSH SENTENCE

Saying that her crime was "roughly akin to distributing cocaine in a schoolyard," a judge sentenced a West St. Paul mother of four to more than two years in prison for her attempt to inject cocaine while giving birth in a hospital delivery room.

Conrad deFiebre, **Star Tribune** of Minneapolis, October 19, 1989

Lastly, the state must set out a definition of behavior which is so wanton in its disregard for human life and safety that persons engaging in it must be held responsible in the criminal courts. I firmly believe criminalization of certain egregious behavior is an absolute requirement to go along with all of the social and medical planning which is also certainly needed.

We acknowledge that education, intervention, and the greater availability of drug treatment facilities for rich and poor alike is important in establishing a long-term solution to this problem. However, we know from our experience as prosecutors and in day-to-day life that people will not always do the right thing for the right reasons. Every day we see persons who know the difference between right and wrong, but who are unwilling to conform their behavior to acceptable standards. Obviously there is no exception in the case of pregnant women.

CRIMINAL SANCTIONS

Practically every high school in this nation has driver education courses, and there is no question that most drivers know the rules of the road. That, however, hasn't solved all of the highway safety problems that this society has encountered over the years. We are still required to conduct arrests of those people who, although knowing of the law, choose to disobey it. The analogy is no less accurate in regard to serious crime in our society, even when committed by drug addicts or pregnant women.

We have decided to continue to play a key role in assisting our legislative leaders to draft appropriate legislation which, through criminal sanctions, discourages individuals from engaging in behavior harmful to the most innocent and defenseless members of our society, the newborn. We also encourage others, including

INCARCERATION

Some judges and prosecutors have been incarcerating pregnant, dope-addicted women as a way to protect both lives at risk. It is, of course, a last-ditch effort to put the force of law between a mother's dangerous, unrehabilitative behavior and the very life of her unborn child.

Peter B. Gemma, Jr., "Threat of Jail Can Cure Junkie Moms", **USA Today,** October 23, 1990

the medical community, to assist the State in formulating and funding programs which will encourage and provide appropriate prenatal care and drug addiction treatment to anyone regardless of economic ability.

Only a comprehensive, well-funded effort which acknowledges the roles of intervention, prevention, education and deterrence can possibly accomplish the objective of guaranteeing the right of our children to a healthy birth.

PREGNANT ADDICTS NEED TREATMENT, NOT PUNISHMENT

American Civil Liberties Union

Kary L. Moss, Esq., is a staff attorney for the Women's Rights Project of the American Civil Liberties Union (ACLU). Lynn M. Palthrow, Esq. is a staff attorney for the Reproductive Freedom Project of the ACLU. And Judy Crockett is a legislative representative for the ACLU. The ACLU is a non-partisan organization with more than 275,000 members devoted to protecting the Bill of Rights.

Points to Consider:

1. What are the shortcomings of existing alcohol and drug treatment programs in helping pregnant addicts?

2. Explain the new crime identified by the ACLU: continuing pregnancy while addicted.

3. What is the effect of prosecutions on the doctor-patient relationship?

4. Why is prosecution of drug-dependent pregnant women contrary to constitutional law, according to the ACLU?

5. Summarize the ACLU's recommendation to the federal government.

Excerpted from testimony by the American Civil Liberties Union before the House Select Committee on Children, Youth and Families, May 17, 1990.

Prosecutions also deter pregnant women from getting what little health care is available.

We are very concerned that alcohol and drug dependent women obtain the prenatal and medical care that they need in order to promote their health and the health of their children. Yet many alcohol and drug treatment programs close their doors to pregnant women. Although many programs were not designed to address the needs of alcohol and drug dependent pregnant women, the programs may provide the only hope, in a given geographic area, for help for these women.

Even where services are available, they are often glaringly insufficient. For example, few provide prenatal care, child care, or other services found essential to successful treatment for women. The National Institute for Drug Abuse recognized over a decade ago that the inability to obtain child care prevents many women from participating in drug treatment programs.

CRIMINAL PROSECUTIONS

The federal government should take steps to stop the trend to subject alcohol and drug dependent women to criminal prosecution for their alcohol or drug use during pregnancy. The American Civil Liberties Union has been involved as counsel or advisor in most of these cases. Our national survey of these prosecutions confirm that women of color, poor women, and battered women are the primary victims. In none of these cases have the men whose violence threatened the health of the fetus been charged with child endangerment.

None of the women arrested were charged with the crime of possession of illegal drugs. Instead, they were arrested for a new and independent crime: continuing their pregnancy while addicted to drugs. Because women are discriminated against in drug treatment programs, and because it is virtually impossible to stop using drugs without help, these prosecutions, in effect, punish women for their decision to continue a pregnancy. These prosecutions thus violate constitutional privacy and liberty guarantees that protect the right to decide "whether to bear or beget a child."

Prosecutions also deter pregnant women from getting what little health care is available. As Senator Herbert Kohl stated at Congressional hearings on perinatal substance abuse, "mothers — afraid of criminal prosecution — fail to seek the very prenatal

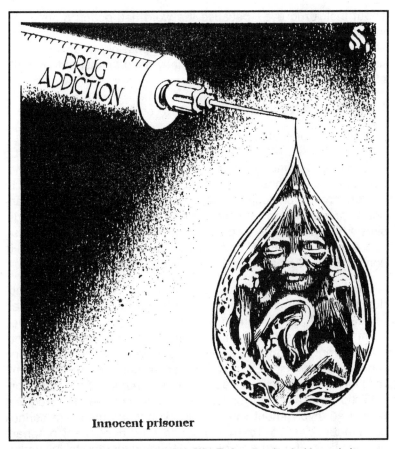

Innocent prisoner

Cartoon by David Seavey. Copyright 1990, **USA Today**. Reprinted with permission.

care that could help their babies and them." Women are also discouraged from seeking help because of the fear that they will lose custody of their children. According to Ricardo Quiroga, who is helping to set up an alcohol recovery house for Hispanic women with children in Massachusetts, women "don't want to seek help for fear they will lose their children."

Prosecutions also undermine doctor-patient trust. Those women who seek medical care are often too frightened to speak openly to their doctors about their alcohol or drug dependency problems. In Florida, for example, after "uniformed officers wearing guns entered Bayfront Medical Center...to investigate new mothers suspected of cocaine abuse," doctors reported that they could no longer "depend on the mothers to tell them the truth about their drug use...because the word had gotten around that the police will have to be notified." Without honest communication between doctor and patient, it will be impossible to provide pregnant women with the medical care they need to ensure the health of the mothers and babies.

UNDERSTANDING

Criminal prosecution, for the "crime" of being alcohol or drug dependent and pregnant reflects a lack of understanding that drug and alcohol dependency is not demonstrative of "willful" behavior but rather, is an illness whose cure has confounded generations of doctors and psychologists. We do not suggest that a woman cannot be prosecuted for a crime, such as possession of illegal drugs, simply because she is pregnant. Rather it is the focus on the drug use during pregnancy, as the basis for the prosecution, that is contrary to well-established principles of constitutional law.

Criminal prosecution is also ultimately premised on the assumption that pregnant addicts are indifferent to the health of their fetuses, or that the women willfully seek to cause their fetuses harm. These assumptions are incorrect: real resource constraints may prevent women from securing treatment or proper care during their pregnancies. Even when women can secure treatment, recovery may be constrained by the very nature of the addiction. Addiction typically involves loss of control over use of a drug and continued involvement with a drug even when there are serious consequences. To treat alcohol and drug dependent pregnant women as indifferent and deliberate wrongdoers is to misunderstand the nature of addiction.

CONSTITUTIONAL RIGHTS

For all of these reasons, the American Civil Liberties Union opposes criminal prosecutions of alcohol or drug dependent women whose only "crime" is choosing to continue a pregnancy. We support a woman's constitutional right to decide whether or not to terminate a pregnancy free of governmental interference or coercion. The federal government should discourage states from enacting laws that would punish alcohol or drug dependent women who continue their pregnancies.

Recently, Oklahoma enacted a law that requires mandatory reporting to social services; if they find evidence of alcohol or drug use, they are authorized to provide that information to district attor-

PREGNANCY AND CRIME

Prosecutions of pregnant women and civil proceedings for removal of newborns cannot rationally be limited to illegal conduct because many activities that are legal can damage developing babies. Women who are diabetic or obese, women with cancer or epilepsy who need drugs that could harm the fetus, and women who are too poor to eat adequately or to get prenatal care could all be characterized as "fetal abusers".

Because no woman can provide the perfect womb, criminal prosecutions come dangerously close to turning pregnancy itself into a crime.

American Civil Liberties Union position paper on Pregnant Women with Drug Addiction Problems, June, 1990

neys. Minnesota has amended its criminal code to mandate reporting of pregnant women who use drugs, the testing of some pregnant women for the presence of drugs, and the testing of newborns for drugs with results reported to Department of Health. Failure to report may be a misdemeanor. Utah now requires medical personnel to report women whose children are born with fetal alcohol syndrome or drug dependency.

These reporting laws harm poor women and women of color the most. One study of Pinnellas County, Florida, for example, conducted by the National Association for Perinatal Addiction Research and Education, found that African-American women were ten times more likely to be reported to child abuse authorities than were white women even though white women were more likely to have used drugs prior to their first visit to the doctor. Researchers surveyed five public health clinics. They found that 14.8 percent of all the women tested positive for alcohol, marijuana, cocaine and/or opiates, with white women 1.09 times more likely to have used alcohol or drugs prior to their first visit to the doctor. Yet, of the 133 pregnant women reported to county health authorities as substance abusers, 85 were African-American and only 45 were white. While we need to undertake similar studies in other geographic areas, there is no reason to believe that Pinnellas County, Florida is not representative of reporting practices throughout the country.

Moreover, it appears from anecdotal evidence that women in government-subsidized facilities are routinely tested for drug use while women who can afford private health care are not tested. Women who cannot afford prenatal care may be labeled "high risk" and tested without their consent, even if their failure to obtain care is the result of poverty. Similarly, hospital practices may vary from area to area. Without standards, hospitals deciding who to report to social services or county attorneys may be improperly influenced by race and class.

LIBERTY AND PRIVACY

Constitutional liberty and privacy guarantees, as well as privacy statutes in some states, however, should prohibit hospitals from revealing patients' medical histories to county prosecutors or social service agencies. The patients' privacy right, defined by the Supreme Court in Whalen v. Roe as "their interest in the nondisclosure of private information and also their interest in making important decisions independently," encompasses a patient's right to nondisclosure of his or her medical history. Medical records are ordinarily entitled to a high degree of protection, and courts have upheld the sanctity of the doctor-patient relationship in the face of threats posed by reporting requirements.

CONCLUSION

Addicts require rehabilitation, not punishment. The federal government should take the initiative on this issue and prohibit the discrimination against alcohol and drug dependent pregnant women in treatment programs and the punishment of women by punitive state laws. In addition, the government should increase the appropriations to local treatment programs to ensure that alcohol and drug dependent pregnant women can obtain comprehensive care during their pregnancy.

CRIME, PREGNANCY AND DRUGS

A CRIMINAL JUSTICE
APPROACH IS JUSTIFIED

Jill Hiatt and Janet Dinsmore

Jill Hiatt is the Senior Attorney at the National Center for Prosecution of Child Abuse and Deputy District Attorney for Alameda County, California. Janet Dinsmore is the Communications Director for the Center and has worked for a variety of children's groups and written extensively on legal and social reform.

Points to Consider:

1. What are the elements in criminal sanction that can effectively reduce drug abuse?

2. Explain how "diversion" works with pregnant, drug-abusing women.

3. According to the authors, what is needed, in addition to extensive support, for successful treatment?

4. What is the "hit bottom syndrome", and why must intervention occur first?

Excerpted from testimony by Jill Hiatt and Janet Dinsmore before the House Select Committee on Children, Youth and Families, May 17, 1990.

***For many people, the alternative to prison will be
the grave.***

On Mother's Day a 28 year-old woman stands in a prison hall-
way holding her child and cries. She is a prisoner and she is having the first visit from her children in 13 months. But the reasons
for her tears appear much greater than the visit alone. It is the
first time, she says, she can hold her children as a drug-free
woman. She credits prison with helping her to "be clean for the
first time since I was 13 years old," and said, "it is a blessing for
me to be here."

With national attention focused on drug use and drug-related
crime and violence, few issues provoke more controversy or frustration than substance abuse by pregnant women. There is little
dispute over its undesirability or harmfulness — to the woman, the
fetus or existing children in the home. But there is intense dis-
agreement over how, when, where and who should attempt to
stop it, and whose rights take precedence.

PREVALENT MYTH

One of the most prevalent myths is that treatment must be voluntary to be effective and that those who abuse drugs would stop
doing so if treatment were available. Given the fact that for many
drug users, arrest is the precipitating factor for their entry into
treatment, this is simply unrealistic. Drug counselors, probation
officers, and former addicts readily acknowledge that court supervision is often critical to maintenance in a treatment program.
Research confirms that while criminal sanctions alone do not
reduce drug abuse, the coercive power, surveillance potential and
time offered through criminal sanctions open significant opportunities for effectively treating the cocaine-heroin abuser...There are a
variety of pressures that bring hardcore drug abusers into treatment: parents, employers, loved ones and friends may all apply
psychological and social pressures. The most powerful pressure,
however, may be the threat of legal sanction — the threat of arrest
and conviction, and most importantly, the threat of incarceration.
The leverage created by this threat, and by the sanction itself, per-
mits treatment to be considered a viable option by serious
abusers.

The fact that treatment counselors, health professionals and former substance abusers acknowledge this fact has not softened

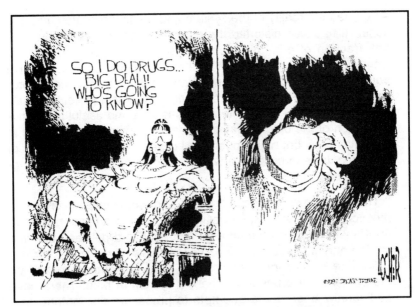

Cartoon by Dick Locher. Reprinted by permission: **Tribune Media Services.**

the outcry against "punitive measures". Is anyone listening?

Realistically, the only way that answers will be found to the complex questions posed by parental drug use is through understanding and cooperation. To gain that cooperation it may be necessary for social service, women's rights and health groups to look more closely at their prejudices and the power and potential for good that exist with the criminal justice system. At the same time, criminal justice professionals may be called on to lay down their spears and look more carefully at the big picture, to see whether traditional forms of law enforcement can be better shaped to deal with a problem that is both legal and social in nature.

One of the largest and most powerful forces in this country is the criminal justice system. One may decry that fact but it is nonetheless so. Since drug use is against the law, the criminal justice system has a powerful tool in its hands. It is time for all concerned groups to find ways of using that tool to deal with a problem that fails to respond to other attempts to ameliorate it.

PROSECUTION

The perception repeated again and again — that the criminal justice system wants only to punish women by putting them in jail

— ignores the reality of the system and stifles the search for solutions. It has also distorted the debate by focusing attention on a tiny fraction of criminal cases involving drug use by pregnant women and child caretakers. Within the criminal justice system's boundaries rest many different means of dealing with crime: probation, diversion, deferred prosecution, treatment in lieu of incarceration, etc. The list of alternatives is long and useful to consider. Much of the outcry against prosecution, however, is rooted in these very few but highly publicized cases involving novel uses of traditional laws to prosecute women who have given birth to drug-affected babies.

The best known of those cases, in Sanford, Florida, involved the prosecution of a woman for delivery of drugs to a minor based on the transfer of drugs through the umbilical cord between the time of birth and cutting of the cord. Other cases have involved prosecuting the mother for possession of illegal substances based on the presence of drugs in the baby's system at birth. There have additionally been some attempts to prosecute the mother on a variety of abuse theories based on the condition of the baby at birth resulting from the mother's ingestion of drugs during pregnancy. Few of these cases have proceeded to trial and only one is currently known to be pending appeal.

Most of these prosecutions are the result of medical workers' frustrations over a mother's production of not one but two, three or ten babies born with the kind of damage that makes their initial weeks and months a living hell and, it appears, probably haunts them for the remainder of their lives, if they survive. While some deride the apparently punitive focus of these prosecutions, one wonders if those same detractors truly believe we must wait until society resolves underlying problems such as poverty, discrimination and hopelessness before responding to the current crisis with all the creativity we can muster.

The vast majority of drug-related cases processed by the criminal justice system have nothing to do with pregnancy. Drug crimes, however, bring into the system hundreds of thousands of mothers and fathers whose substance abuse endangers their current and future families. It is on these individuals who are already in the system that we should be concentrating our attention. The potential for making a significant impact in terms of successful drug treatment is truly enormous.

PREGNANCY & CRIMINAL BEHAVIOR

Pregnancy does not excuse criminal behavior but in many cases can be an additional factor in assessing an individual's criminal penalty. The use of diversion for example, has long been a means of dealing with drug addicts as well as other first-time criminal offenders. It is similar to probation in that there are requirements that the diverted individual must fulfill but there need be no conviction. If the individual completes diversion requirements, the case is dismissed. At least two diversion programs in the country have been specifically developed for pregnant drug-abusing women, and include such requirements as regular prenatal care and staying off drugs. One program requires participation in a treatment program, and the other strongly encourages it. While these programs are in the very early stages, they seem to hold promise for wide replication in the future.

Most jurisdictions grant probation in many cases involving pregnant drug abusers. Probation can and should include not only drug treatment but also a requirement that the women participate in a prenatal program that will help keep her and the baby healthy. In some cases when the crime is either so serious or is a repeat offense the court can and often does sentence drug offenders to treatment facilities in lieu of jail. Such sentences can benefit both baby and mother, allowing the baby a drug-free prenatal environment and the hope that the mother will remain drug-free following completion of her sentence.

When all else fails and there is no alternative to incarceration, comprehensive long-term drug treatment in jail or prison should be used. Even here, significant incentives for treatment can be built in through early release programs based on credits earned through participation in drug treatment. The inclusion of such treatment within institutions is becoming more common with the rising recognition of the close relationships between criminal behavior and drug use.

TREATMENT

Prosecutors throughout the country acknowledge the lack of effective treatment facilities and in many jurisdictions are working with other agencies to identify funding and comprehensive programs for pregnant addicts. The National Center for Prosecution of Child Abuse receives many calls from prosecutors who are working with the task forces made up of health, social service, family court and law enforcement officials to develop services for drug-ravaged families. The National District Attorneys' Association (NDAA) has also formally recommended a treatment option for offenders on probation and a method for funding drug abuse education and treatment in its "Proposed Amendments to the Uniform Controlled Substances Act" (UCSA, 1989). NDAA has also proposed in the UCSA a funding mechanism that has raised millions of dollars for drug education and treatment in New Jersey.

There is much discussion of the need for treatment that is accessible, that accepts pregnant women on Medicaid, that offers resources for residential or day care if needed, and that is sensitive to the unique needs of female addicts and women of color. What is missing from the discussion is recognition that many addicts — particularly crack addicts who face a long-term recovery period — find it difficult or impossible to remain drug-free without some outside coercion in addition to extensive support. At a recent meeting of the coalition on Alcohol and Drug Dependent Women and Their Children, a veteran Philadelphia health worker, Bruni Sepulvada, spoke eloquently of the problems she faces in persuading addicts to get into and remain committed to treatment. Despite apparently heroic efforts on the part of her health workers, the work is filled with frustration and failure. One of the bright spots, she said, is a successful "behavior modification" program involving hard-core parolees whose requirements include participation in treatment. Several, she said, have asked to remain under electronic surveillance past their release date, knowing they could resist street pressures to resume drug use only when they and their peers knew they had to answer to the criminal justice system.

CRIMINAL JUSTICE SYSTEM

According to the *New York Times*, 40-60 percent of the children entering kindergarten in some neighborhoods have drug-related problems. Last year's jump in child abuse and neglect reports — reaching an all-time high of 2.4 million — were directly related to parental and caretaker drug use, according to the National Committee for Prevention of Child Abuse. The Committee also reported that child protection agencies were so overwhelmed with cases, only the most severe were being addressed, leaving others to worsen until they too became emergencies.

Alcoholics Anonymous, one of the most respected and successful addiction treatment programs, has said that people do not seek treatment before "hitting bottom". Those who would remove intervention by the criminal justice system as a "bottom" ignore the fact that for many people, the alternative to prison will be the grave. There is no time left to wait for the "hit bottom syndrome" to occur naturally to help save the women and children that drugs are destroying. The criminal justice system, working in partnership with other agencies, has the tools to force the acceptance of treatment now, and ways must be found to work together with rather than against each other.

The woman being visited by her children in prison paid a high price for her habit but the result is beyond value. In exchange for some months in prison, she got back a life, one that had been in limbo for 15 years. Equally important, her children gained a mother they would never have known otherwise. She apparently believes it was well worth the price.

So perhaps it is time for the criminal justice system, social services, and woman's rights groups to sit down and talk, and start acting together on behalf of those who need true advocacy. Only as a joint effort will this tragic problem be solved, and it is one problem we have to solve.

23   CRIME, PREGNANCY AND DRUGS

PUNITIVE ACTIONS
WILL NOT WORK

Allan I. Trachtenberg

Alan I. Trachtenberg, M.D., M.P.H., is the Medical Director of Bay Area Addiction Research and Treatment (BAART) and the Family Addiction Center for Education and Treatment (FACET) in Berkeley, California.

Points to Consider:

1. How might fear of prosecution contribute to an increase in newborn disability?

2. How might the women addict be helped before she conceives?

3. In what way might tobacco be viewed as more dangerous to babies than cocaine?

4. What barriers to treatment exist, and how might they be removed?

Excerpted from testimony by Allan I. Trachtenberg before the House Select Committee on Children, Youth and Families, April 19, 1990.

Fear of prosecution will not scare pregnant addicts out of using drugs.

I would like to make three essential points today.

The first is that pregnant and non-pregnant addicted women desperately need increased access to appropriate medical and supportive services. They can ill afford increased barriers like the fear of prosecution or the disdainful attitude of many professionals. It would be a far better use of scarce funds to allocate them to our starved treatment infrastructure than to the already overburdened judicial system.

The second point is that addiction, along with many other diseases, is a public health consequence of oppression and poverty. I initially realized this while I was serving in the United States Public Health Service on the Pine Ridge Indian Reservation. This was the first time I came face-to-face with a people who had been nearly decimated by long term social neglect and the consequent problems of intergenerational poverty, much as the population of our inner cities. The current epidemic of drug addiction is growing up like weeds on a neglected lawn. The real solution is not toxic herbicides, nor is it cost effective to pull each weed out by the roots. The real solution is to seed and water the lawn.

The third point addresses our hysterical and judgmental attitudes about drug addiction, which is a chronic relapsing disease that is seldom cured, but for which some effective treatments do exist. As a society we are currently focusing an inordinate amount of attention on particular illicit drugs and virtually ignoring other much more important detriments to the health of our women and children, such as cigarette smoking and the lack of universal access to medical care.

ACCESS AND BARRIERS TO CARE

To return to my first point, I would plead to this committee to stop the obstetrical wards of this country from being turned into obstetrical jails. My patients are surprisingly good at staying away from jail situations. A policy that drives any population away from prenatal care decreases that population's birthweight and increases the amount of disability and death which will occur in the newborns of that population. Addiction is defined as a disease of compulsive substance abuse which the addict continues despite adverse consequences. Fear of prosecution will not scare preg-

145

TREATMENT

While there is some truth to all stereotypes, not all women who use drugs during pregnancy lack concern for their child. Rehabilitation services for pregnant women are often not available, and as a result, many women who want drug treatment cannot get it. When such services are available, women are able to recover from their addiction.

Iris E. Smith, M.P.H., Laboratory of Human and Behavior Genetics, Emory University, in testimony before the **House Select Committee on Children, Youth and Families,** April 19, 1990

nant addicts out of using drugs; it will just scare them away from any contact with a system that they must access to get the prenatal care and drug treatment that they so desperately need. Even if a woman continues to use drugs during pregnancy, proper prenatal care will still improve the birth outcome in comparison to a drug using woman who obtains no prenatal care.

The physician who cares for a pregnant addict has several patients. We care for the woman, we care for the unborn, we care for the already born (her other children) and we care for the father, if he is present. These are fragile families that, if given proper support, could in many cases be better environments for children than our chaotic foster care system. Make no mistake, there are certainly cases in which children do need to be removed from the biological family. But the judicial approach should be a last resort, only after treatment has been available and failed or not been utilized despite its geographic and cultural accessibility.

THE ROOTS AND BITTER FRUITS OF ADDICTION

My second point addresses drug addiction as a public health consequence of oppression and poverty. Most of my female patients have been either sexually or physically abused as children or severely assaulted as adults. Many are forced by the economic circumstances of their lives to exchange sexual behaviors for the means they depend on to survive.

Most influential people in our society seem to have little interest in an addicted woman until she becomes pregnant, often unintentionally. Then, if she doesn't happen to live in one of the few states whose Medicaid programs still cover abortion services, and if she cannot accumulate enough money in a limited time, she may be unable to terminate her pregnancy despite her wish to do so. Whether or not the pregnancy was desired, many programs will not admit or continue to treat pregnant clients for various reasons. These may include the additional and often unreimbursed cost of the extra services and monitoring required during pregnancy. After delivery, society again loses interest in the woman, except in her role as a potentially unfit mother.

If we want to create good environments for the children of addicted mothers, we must consider making the resources available for safe and healthy homes. Then none of my patients would ever again have to resort to prostitution to avoid living on the street. Pregnancy and childbirth have been shown to be risk factors for homelessness. In a caring society this should not be the case.

But why are we focusing today on the pregnant addict? Does anyone care about the addict before she conceives? Who cares enough about her to fund the non-threatening contraceptive services she may need to keep from getting pregnant and to keep from getting sexually transmitted diseases like AIDS or cancer of the cervix?

Although many of the pregnancies we see are unintentional, some are very much desired by the patients. We must recognize that reproduction may be the only source of self-esteem available to these marginalized women who are given the clear message from our society that they are not worthy of concern or protection.

DRUGS & DISEASE

In an effort to provide what seemed to be a solution to the last epidemic of heroin addiction, many state legislatures made the non-medical possession of injection equipment ("works") illegal. The consequence of this legislation, now as apparent to many addicts as it is to the public health community, was to greatly increase the transmission of bloodborne infections such as hepatitis B and HIV from addict to addict. From addicts these infections spread to their sex partners and children.

Legislators must recognize that many of the diseases associated with drug addiction are not the result of the drugs themselves but rather of the social environment in which the drugs are ingested. A good example of this is the epidemic of tuberculosis now being seen in the young adult crack smokers of Contra Costa County. People smoke crack in crowded rooms with ventilation purposely minimized to lessen their risk of detection. They inhale hot gases and cough in close quarters, creating an environment practically tailor-made for optimal transmission of the tubercle bacillus. One or two people in this environment may have had TB infections for many years, until their more recent and probably unsuspected HIV infections broke down their immunity. Pulmonary tuberculosis will likely go undetected for some time, since addicts are even more likely than non-addicts to ignore symptoms such as cough and weight loss. Meanwhile they spread their TB infection by the respiratory route. Luckily some of these crack addicts will also be addicted to heroin, and some of them will find their way into one of our clinics where we perform skin testing for TB infection on all of our patients. We work closely with the county health department to eradicate this preventable disease.

A PUBLIC HEALTH PERSPECTIVE BEYOND THE STEREOTYPES

My third point has to do with the hysteria with which America is now addressing the problem of addiction to illicit drugs. The news media barrage us with story after story of the alternating waves of stimulant and opiate addiction which have swept this country since the early part of this century. But why are we focusing only on illicit drugs? Legal drugs like tobacco are causing vastly more disability and death to America's newborns than heroin and cocaine. Should we imprison pregnant smokers? Should we continue to give federal subsidies to a tobacco industry that addicts thousands of future mothers every year with cynical advertising campaigns to convince teenage girls they will be sexier and have more fun if they smoke this or that brand of cigarette? At least five to ten percent of all stillbirths and neonatal deaths are attributable to smoking in pregnancy. Furthermore, pregnancies of smoking mothers show about the same increased risk of infant wastage as pregnancies at high altitudes.

Would this committee be prepared to follow a proposed policy for jailing pregnant addicts (for the protection of the unborn) to its logical conclusion by recommending that all pregnant women who stubbornly remain in high altitude domiciles should be forcibly detained in sea-level, smoke-free, prenatal camps? I do not advocate such action. However, across the U.S. at least 18% of all low birth weight is caused by smoking, while even in Alameda County, California, which contains inner city Oakland neighborhoods decimated by crack, only 10% of the low birth weight in babies born to black women is attributable to cocaine.

RECOMMENDATIONS

What solutions can I recommend to the committee? I have three general recommendations: 1) Decrease the barriers to treatment, 2) Decrease the stigma of being in treatment, and 3) Decrease the need for treatment.

To decrease barriers to needed treatment:

a) Treatment in all modalities medically established to be useful in the management of drug addiction should be made available in all localities.

b) A full spectrum of primary care services including child care, should be funded and available in all drug treatment clinics, so that the addicted mother with children and no working automobile can do "One stop shopping".

c) Travel vouchers or other transportation assistance should be readily available to all pregnant women, especially pregnant addicts, for whom a car breakdown can lead to a catastrophe.

To decrease the need for drug treatment we must decrease the risk factors for drug abuse and addiction. The most important risk factor for drug addiction in America today is poverty. How will we create social structures that give other options to oppressed and despairing women besides the exchange of sexual behaviors for money and the use of illicit drugs for relief from the emotional pain of their day-to-day existence? I believe that we must create economic options for young adults in the inner cities and on the reservations that will provide alternative means of sustenance and self-esteem. Then, when they are offered a role in the seductive drug economy, be it as a supplier or a consumer, they will know that they do have something to lose by taking that first step. Maybe then they will be able to "Just say no."

WHAT IS POLITICAL BIAS?

This activity may be used as an individualized study guide for students in libraries and resource centers or as a discussion catalyst in small group and classroom discussions.

Many readers are unaware that written material usually expresses an opinion or bias. The skill to read with insight and understanding requires the ability to detect different kinds of bias. **Political bias, race bias, sex bias, ethnocentric bias** and **religious bias** are five basic kinds of opinions expressed in editorials and literature that attempt to persuade. This activity will focus on political bias defined in the glossary below.

FIVE KINDS OF EDITORIAL OPINION OR BIAS

Sex Bias — the expression of dislike for and/or feeling of superiority over a person because of gender or sexual preference

Race Bias — the expression of dislike for and/or feeling of superiority over a racial group

Ethnocentric Bias — the expression of a belief that one's own group, race, religion, culture or nation is superior
Ethnocentric persons judge others by their own standards and values.

Political Bias — the expression of opinions and attitudes about government-related issues on the local, state, national or international level

Religious Bias — the expression of a religious belief or attitude

---

Guidelines

Read through the following statements and decide which ones represent political opinion or bias. Evaluate each statement by using the method indicated below.

- **Mark (P) for any statements that reflect political opinion or bias.**

- **Mark (F) for any factual statements.**

- **Mark (O) for any statements of opinion that reflect other kinds of opinion or bias.**

- **Mark (N) for any statements that you are not sure about.**

_____1. The most important risk factor for drug addiction today is poverty.

_____2. Many drug and alcohol programs do not address the needs of drug dependent pregnant women.

_____3. Not all women who use drugs during pregnancy have a lack of concern for their child.

_____4. The problem of children born either exposed or addicted to alcohol or drugs has become a difficult issue in every city and state.

_____5. Fear of prosecution will not scare pregnant addicts out of using drugs.

_____6. A few states have amended their neglect, abuse and termination of parental rights laws to make earlier removal easier.

_____7. Pregnant addicts who cannot kick the habit should be required to enter treatment programs upon giving birth to a drug-exposed infant.

_____8. It is difficult to draft a provision that accurately reflects the scientific basis for a positive drug test.

_____9. Throughout the country there is a lack of funding and comprehensive programs for pregnant addicts.

_____10. No subject is more charged with emotion than the decision to remove children from their home.

_____11. Criminal prosecution is ultimately premised on the assumption that pregnant addicts are indifferent to the health of their fetuses.

_____12. Prosecutions deter pregnant women from getting what little health care is available.

_____13. States have reacted very cautiously to the approach of controlling the mother's behavior through criminal laws.

_____14. The federal government should take steps to prosecute women who use drugs or alcohol during pregnancy.

_____15. Lack of child care is a major factor in drug care which prevents many women from getting help.

Other Activities

1. Locate three examples of political opinion or bias in the readings from Chapter Four.

2. Make up one-sentence statements that would be an example of each of the following: **sex bias, race bias, ethnocentric bias, and religious bias.**

APPENDIX

Organizations and Information

National Resource Centers:

The Clearinghouse for Drug Exposed Children
Division of Behavioral and Developmental Pediatrics
University of California, San Francisco
400 Parnassus Avenue, Room A203
San Francisco, CA 94143-0314
Telephone: (415) 476-9691

National Clearinghouse for Alcohol and Drug Information
P.O. Box 2345
Rockville, MD 20852
Telephone: (301) 468-2600
Toll free: 1-(800) 729-6686

NAPARE
National Association for Perinatal Addiction Research and
Education
11 E. Hubbard Street, Suite 200
Chicago, IL 60611
Telephone: (312) 329-9131
Toll free: NAPARE Alcohol, Drugs and Pregnancy Helpline:
1-(800) 638-2229

National Council on Alcoholism and Drug Dependence
12 West 21 Street
New York, NY 10010
Telephone: (212) 206-6770
Toll free Helpline: 1-(800) 622-2255 or 1-(800) 475-4673

National Perinatal Information Center
One State Street, Suite 102
Providence, RI 02908
Telephone: (401) 274-0650

National Association for Native American Children of Alcoholics
P.O. Box 18736
Seattle, WA 98118
Telephone: (206) 322-5601

National Black Alcoholism Council
1629 K Street, NW, Suite 802
Washington, DC 20006
Telephone: (202) 296-2696

National Coalition for Hispanic Health & Human Services
1030 15th Street, NW, Suite 1035
Washington, DC 20005
Telephone: (202) 371-2100

Centers for Disease Control (CDC)
National Center for Environmental Health (NCEH)
1600 Clifton Road
Mailstop F-29
Atlanta, GA 30333
Telephone: (404) 488-7370

National Organization on Fetal Alcohol Syndrome (NOFAS)
1815 H Street, NW, Suite 750
Washington, DC 20006
Telephone: (202) 785-4585
Toll free: 1-(800) 66-NOFAS (1-800-666-6327)

National Indian Board on Alcohol and Drug Abuse
P.O. Box 8
Turtle Lake, WI 54889

BIBLIOGRAPHY

General References

Burch, M.R. "Behavioral Treatment of Drug Exposed Infants: Analyzing and Treating Aggression." **Children Today** 1992: 12-15.

Gregorchik, L.A. "The Cocaine-exposed Children Are Here." **Phi Delta Kappan** May 1992: 709-711.

Griffith, D.R. "Prenatal Exposure to Cocaine and Other Drugs: Developmental and Educational Prognoses." **Phi Delta Kappan** Sept. 1992: 30-4.

Maddux, B.K. "Mother Love." **Life** May 1992: 49-53+.

"Newborns and Addiction." **Newsweek** 20 Apr. 1992: 75.

Sautter, R.C. "Crack: Healing the Children." **Phi Delta Kappan** Nov. 1992: K1-K10.

Sullum, J. "The Cocaine Kids." **Reason** Aug./Sept. 1992: 14.

Tyler, R. "Prenatal Drug Exposure: An Overview of Associated Problems and Intervention Strategies." **Phi Delta Kappan** May 1992: 705-708.

Scholarly References

Abma, Joyce C., and Frank L. Mott. "Substance Use and Prenatal Care During Pregnancy Among Young Women." **Family Planning Perspectives** May-June 1991: 23, 3, 117-122, 128.

Besharov, Douglas J. "The Children of Crack: Will We Protect Them?" **Public Welfare** Fall 1989: 47, 4, 6-11.

Burch, Mary R. "Behavioral Treatment of Drug Exposed Infants: Analyzing and Treating Aggression." **Children Today** 1992: v. 21, n. 1, 12-15.

Chang, Grace; Carroll, Kathleen M.; Behr, Heidi M.; and Kosten, Thomas R. "Improving Treatment Outcome in Pregnant Opiate-Dependent Women." **Journal of Substance Abuse Treatment** Fall 1992: 9, 4, 327-330.

Coles, C.D.; Smith, I.; Fernhoff, P.M.; and Falek. "Neonatal Neurobehavioral Characteristics as Correlates of Maternal Alcohol Use During Gestation." **Alcoholism: Clinical and Experimental Research** 1985: 9(5), 454-460.

Donoghoe, Martin C. "Sex, HIV and the Injecting Drug User." **British Journal of Addiction** Mar. 1992: 87, 3, 405-416.

Donovan, C.L. "Factors Predisposing, Enabling, and Reinforcing Routine Screening of Patients for Preventing Fetal Alcohol Syndrome: A Survey of New Jersey Physicians." **Journal of Drug Education** 1991: 21(1), 35-42.

Dorczak, Anita, and T. Brettel Dawson. "Unborn Child Abuse: Contemplating Legal Solution." **Canadian Journal of Family Law/Revue Canadienne de Droit Familial** Spring 1991: 9, 2, 133-156.

Eliason, M.J., and J.K. Williams. "Fetal Alcohol Syndrome and the Neonate." **Journal of Perinatal and Neonatal Nursing** April 1990: 3(4), 64-72.

Elliot, D.J., and N. Johnson. "Fetal Alcohol Syndrome: Implications and Counseling Considerations." **Personnel and Guidance Journal** 1983: 62(2), 67-69.

Ernhart, C.B.; Morrow-Tlucak, M.; Sokol, R.J.; and Martier, S. "Underreporting of Alcohol Use in Pregnancy." **Alcoholism: Clinical and Experimental Research** 1988: 12(4), 506-511.

Farrell, Michael, and John Strang. "Substance Use and Misuse in Childhood and Adolescence." **Journal of Child Psychology and Psychiatry and Allied Disciplines** Jan. 1991: 32, 1, 109-128.

Flannery, Michael T. "Court Ordered Prenatal Intervention: A Final Means to the End of Gestational Substance Abuse." **Journal of Family Law** May 1991-1992: 30, 3, 519-604.

Fullilove, Mindy Thompson; Lown, E. Anne; and Fullilove, Robert E. "Crack'hos and Skeezers: Traumatic Experiences of Women Crack Users." **Journal of Sex Research** May 1992: 9, 2, 275-267.

Gaines, Judith, and Stephen R. Kandall. "Counseling Issues Related to Maternal Substance Abuse and Subsequent Sudden Infant Death Syndrome in Offspring." **Clinical Social Work Journal** Summer 1992: 20, 2, 169-177.

Greene, Dwight L. "Abusive Prosecutors: Gender, Race and Class Discretion and the Prosecution of Drug-Addicted Mothers." **Buffalo Law Review** Fall 1991: 39, 3, 737-802.

Gustavsson, Nora S. "Drug Exposed Infants and Their Mothers: Facts, Myths, and Needs." **Social Work in Health Care** 1992: 16, 4, 87-100.

Hanson, J.W. "Preventing the Fetal Alcohol Syndrome." **The Female Patient** Oct. 1979: 38-41, 44.

Harrison, Michelle. "Drug Addiction in Pregnancy: The Interface of Science, Emotion, and Social Policy." **Journal of Substance Abuse Treatment** 1991: 8, 4, 261-268.

Horowitz, R. "A Coordinated Public Health and Child Welfare Response to Perinatal Substance Abuse." **Children Today** 1990: 19(4), 8-12.

Kaskutas, Lee, and Thomas K. Greenfield. "First Effects of Warning Labels on Alcoholic Beverage Containers." **Drug and Alcohol Dependence** Oct. 1992: 31, 1, 1-14.

Kelley, Susan J. "Parenting Stress and Child Maltreatment in Drug-Exposed Children." **Child Abuse and Neglect** 1992: 16, 3, 317-328.

Keyes, Lisa Janovy. "Rethinking the Aim of the 'War on Drugs': States' Roles in Preventing Substance Abuse by Pregnant Women." **Wisconsin Law Review** 1992: 1, 197-232.

King, Patricia A. "Helping Women Helping Children: Drug Policy and Future Generations." **Milbank Quarterly** 1991: 69, 4, 595-621.

Kirp, David L. "The Pitfalls of Fetal Protection." **Society** Mar.-Apr. 1991: 28, 3(191), 70-76.

Lamanna, M.L. "Alcohol Related Birth Defects: Implications for Education." **Journal of Drug Education** 1982: 12(2), 113-123.

Maher, Lisa. "Punishment and Welfare: Crack Cocaine and the Regulation of Mothering." **Women and Criminal Justice** 1992: 3, 2, 35-70.

Maher, Lisa. "Criminalizing Pregnancy — The Downside of a Kinder, Gentler Nation?" **Social Justice** Fall 1990: 17, 3, 111-135.

May, P.A. "Alcohol and Drug Misuse Prevention Programs for American Indians: Needs and Opportunities." **Journal of Studies on Alcohol** 1986: 47(3), 137-195.

May, P.A., and K.J. Hymbaugh. "A Macro-Level Fetal Alcohol Syndrome Prevention Program for Native Americans and Alaska Natives: Description and Evaluation." **Journal of Studies on Alcohol** 1989: 50(6), 508-518.

May, P.A.; Hymbaugh, K.J.; Aase, J.M.; and Samet, J.M. "Epidemiology of Fetal Alcohol Syndrome Among American Indians of the Southwest." **Social Biology** 1983: 30(4), 374-387.

Melneck, M.J. "Fetal alcohol syndrome: Any Woman Who Drinks Any Amount During Pregnancy Exposes Her Baby to Unnecessary Risks." **Childbirth Educator** Winter 1984: 47-52.

Miller, Suzanne M. "Policy Options: Early Intervention Services for Substance-Exposed Infants." **Journal of Drug Education** 1992: v. 22, n. 4, 273-81.

Raskin, Robert, and Others. "Drug Culture Expertise and Substance Use." **Journal of Youth and Adolescence** Oct. 1992: v. 21, n. 5, 625-37.

Schedler, George. "Forcing Pregnant Drug Addicts to Abort: Rights-Based and Utilitarian Justifications." **Social Theory and Practice** Fall 1992: 18, 3, 347-358.

Serdula, M. et al. "Trends in Alcohol Consumption by Pregnant Women." **Journal of the American Medical Association** Feb. 1991: 265(7), 876-879.

Shoaee, S. "Women and Alcoholism in America: Policy Analysis and Gender-Related Issues." **Future Choices: Toward a National Youth Policy** 1990: 2(2), 9-28.

Smart, Reginald G. "Crack Cocaine Use: A Review of Prevalence & Adverse Effects." **American Journal of Drug and Alcohol Abuse** Mar. 1991: 17, 1, 13-26.

Smith, Iris E.; Dent, Donna Z.; Coles, Claire D.; and Falek, Arthur. "A Comparison Study of Treated and Untreated Pregnant and Postpartum Cocaine-Abusing Women." **Journal of Substance Abuse Treatment** Fall 1992: 9, 4, 343-348.

Smith, I.S., and C.D. Coles. "Multilevel Intervention for Prevention of FAS and Effects of Prenatal Alcohol Exposure." In M. Galater (Ed.), **Recent Developments in Alcoholism Treatment Issues** 1990: v. 9.

Sokol, R.J.; Martier, S.S.; and Ager, J.W. "The T-ACE Questions: Practical Prenatal Detection of Risk-Drinking." **American Journal of Obstetrics and Gynecology** 1989: 160, 863-870.

Solomon, Renee I. "Future Fear: Prenatal Duties Imposed by Private Parties." **American Journal of Law and Medicine** Winter, 1991: 17, 4, 411-434.

Steinmetz, G. "The Preventable Tragedy: Fetal Alcohol Syndrome." **National Geographic** Feb. 1992: 36-39.

Thombs, Dennis L., and Others. "Effects of Social Context and Gender on Drinking Patterns of Young Adults." **Journal of Counseling Psychology** Jan. 1993: v. 40, n. 1, 115-19.

van Dyke, D.C.; Mackay, L.; Ziaylek, E.N. "Management of Severe Feeding Dysfunction in Children with Fetal Alcohol Syndrome." **Clinical Pediatrics** 1982: 21(6), 336-339.

Viadero, D. "Drug-Exposed Children Present Special Problems." **Education Week** Oct. 1989: 1, 10-11.

Weiner, L. and G. Larsson. "Clinical Prevention of Fetal Alcohol Effects: A Reality." **Alcohol Health & Research World** Summer, 1987: 60-63, 92-93.

Willims, G.D.; Stinson, F.S.; Parker, D.A.; Harford, T.C.; Noble, J. "Demographic Trends, Alcohol Abuse and Alcoholism." **Alcohol Health and Research World** 1987: 11(3), 80-83, 91.